Donald W. Pfaff

Estrogens and Brain Function

Neural Analysis of a Hormone-Controlled
Mammalian Reproductive Behavior

With 109 Figures

Springer-Verlag
New York   Heidelberg   Berlin

DONALD W. PFAFF
Professor of Neurobiology and Behavior
The Rockefeller University
New York, New York 10021
USA

Library of Congress Cataloging in Publication Data
Pfaff, Donald W
   Estrogens and brain function.
   Includes index.
   1. Reproduction.   2.   Estrogen—Physiological effect.
3.   Sexual behavior in animals.   4.   Mammals—Behavior.
I.   Title.   [DNLM: 1.   Estrogens—Physiology.   2.   Brain—
Physiology.   3.   Sex behavior, Animal.   4.   Posture.
5.   Mammals.   6.   Reproduction.   QL761 P5 23e]
QP251.P47   599.01'6   80-11900

9 8 7 6 5 4 3 2 1

ISBN 0-387-90487-5 Springer-Verlag New York Heidelberg Berlin
ISBN 3-540-90487-5 Springer-Verlag Berlin Heidelberg New York

Preface

This book brings together some of the results and ideas produced by a large number of people—colleagues and students with whom I am privileged to work in the laboratory at Rockefeller University. In terms of my personal history I see it as a confluence of creative forces—persons from whom I have learned. I was instructed in neuroanatomy by Walle J. H. Nauta at M.I.T., and later in a course at Harvard Medical School under the direction of Richard Sidman. At Harvard Medical School, where M.I.T. graduate students were allowed to cross register, the superb neurophysiology course was under the guiding spirit of Stephen Kuffler. Later, I benefited greatly from participating in his summer course in electrophysiological techniques at Woods Hole. Eric Kandel and his colleagues have provided us with the most exciting contemporary approach to the conceptualization and study of cellular mechanisms for behavior. Here at Rockefeller, Carl Pfaffmann and Neal Miller have been leaders in every sense of the word. Not only did they provide me with opportunities to grow to scientific maturity; they also set an example of clear thinking about mechanisms for mammalian behavior patterns.

I wrote this book to show how the systematic use of increasingly detailed electrophysiological, neuroanatomical, and neuroendocrine techniques can explain the mechanism for a mammalian behavioral response. The behavior in question happens to be sensitive to steroid hormones and plays a central role in reproduction. The writing is intended to be clear enough to enable any person who enjoys *Scientific American* or *Nature* to understand the main lines of data presentation and thought. The presentation is also precise enough that trained researchers and students who can detect gaps or shortcomings may be encouraged to fill them by doing new experiments.

Rockefeller University   DONALD W. PFAFF
New York
January 1980

Contents

Chapter 3

Primary Sensory Neurons

Chapter 4

Spinal Interneurons

Chapter 5

Ascending Neural Pathways

Part 2

Facilitating the Behavior: Sex Hormones in the Brain

Chapter 11

Motoneurons and Response Execution

Part 4

Building on this Paradigm

Chapter 12

Logical and Heuristic Developments

Chapter 13

Summary

Chapter 14

Epilogue

Chapter 1
Introduction

A.   Approaching the Neural Mechanisms of Behavior

Those who study the nervous sytem ultimately aim to explain behavior. They intend to demonstrate how behavioral responses are produced as a function of nerve cell activity. However, even for small bits of neural tissue and restricted forms of behavior, the numbers of nerve cells to be considered are so large and their connections so complex that all sorts of explanatory hypotheses can be imagined. As a result, in the history of neural and behavioral studies, many thinkers have felt free to "neurologize." They could speculate broadly about the overall "organization of the brain" and the control of behavior because, virtually always, the number of facts available to rule out their hypotheses was small. No comprehensive model or hypothesis could be shown to be better than others.

It has therefore been necessary to choose a behavioral problem for which it would be fruitful to gather a great number of behavioral, neuroanatomical, and neurophysiological facts that may be used to narrow down the allowable hypotheses to a small number. With enough of these relevant facts brought to bear, the logical scientific procedure of strong inference (Platt, 1964) can be used to arrive at satisfactory models and hypotheses. In turn, principles can be stated clearly and tested.

This approach discourages the practice of concentrating on a single region of neural tissue, doing a great deal of experimental work on that region, and asking the question, "What does this tissue do?" One does not take a single experimental technique and apply it to all neural tissue and functional problems available. Rather, the objective is to try to see how the nervous system accomplishes a particular "job": that is, we choose a particular pattern of adaptive behavior and investigate how the nervous system produces and controls that behavior. From this information, principles of the neural control of behavior may be induced, and eventually tested with other behavior patterns.

In view of the large number of possible neural mechanisms, we gain advantage by learning as much as possible about a particular behavior pattern. The more facts we have about the behavior itself, the better "fix" we have on the neural mechanism. Thus, it is useful to devote detailed studies to the sensory and motor aspects of the behavior pattern selected (see Section D). Studying the hormonal determinants of the behavior also helps. Knowledge of the sensory and motor facts enables one to study the spinal mechanisms that execute the behavior and, in turn, the brainstem mechanisms that link the spinal neurons to the forebrain. The endocrine data make it easier to study forebrain, especially hypothalamic, circuitry. In general, faced with the complexity of the mammalian central nervous system, we have adopted the strategy of approaching the complete neural mechanism step by step, working from the known to the unknown, and, where possible, moving from the anatomically simple toward the anatomically complex.

B. Old Questions, New Tools

With the "new reflexology" approach, we use the methods of modern neuroanatomy, neurophysiology, and neuroendocrinology to study systematically the neural mechanism for an individual behavior pattern. For instance, we can regard mating behavior responses as hormone-sensitive reflexes (Pfaff, Lewis, Diakow, and Keiner, 1972). Using the term *reflex* in this way does not imply a simple equivalence with the phrase *spinal reflex* or *reflex dependent solely on spinal tissue,* even if the behavior involved partly depends on spinal mechanisms (as mating behavior responses clearly do). We use the term *reflex* to mean that a well-defined set of stimuli reliably determines a well-defined constellation of muscular responses.

Lacking a clear alternative, and driven by the demand for clear deterministic thinking, we use the paradigm of classical reflex physiology for the modern dissection of behavioral mechanisms. Indeed, an important tradition in the history of brain research has been to regard reflex action as a prototype for the study of animal behavior (Fearing, 1930). For instance, in his pioneer attempt to put the study of behavior on a scientific basis (ultimately to link it with the physical sciences) Loeb (1912) said the following:

> It is probably unnecessary to emphasize the fact that it is better for the progress of science to derive the more complex phenomena from simpler components than to do the contrary. For all explanations consist solely in the presentation of a phenomenon as an unequivocal function of the variables by which it is determined . . .The progress of natural science depends upon the

discovery of rationalistic elements or simple natural laws . . . tropisms and tropism-like reactions are elements which pave the way for a rationalistic conception of the psychological reactions of animals. (pp. 58–60)

The understanding of complicated phenomena depends upon an analysis by which they are resolved to their simple elementary components. If we ask what the elementary components are in the physiology of the central nervous system, our attention is directed to a class of processes which are called reflexes. There has been a growing tendency in physiology to make reflexes the basis of the analysis of the functions of the central nervous system. (p. 65; cf. Loeb, 1899)

Sherrington (1906) felt that, aside from questions of volitional control, the study of reflex action could account for the integrated, coordinated flow of behavioral responses:

The study of reflexes as adapted reactions evidently, therefore, includes the actions of two ranks. With the nervous system intact, the reactions of the various parts of that system, the simple reflexes, are ever combined to create unitary harmonies; actions which in their sequence one upon another constitute in their continuity what may be termed the behavior of the individual as a whole. (p. 238)

William James (1890) guessed that even complex behavioral acts, at least in many aspects, might conform to rules based on the study of reflex actions:

In the "loop-line" along which the memories and ideas of the distant are supposed to lie, the action, so far as it is a physical process, must be interpreted after the type of the action in the lower centers. If regarded here as a reflex process, it must be reflex there as well. The current in both places runs out into the muscles only after it has first run in; but while the path by which it runs out is determined in the lower centers by reflexions and fixed among the cell arrangements, in the hemispheres the reflexions are many and instable. This, it will be seen, is only a difference of degree, not of kind, and does not change the reflex type. The conception of *all* action as conforming to this type is the fundamental conception of modern nerve-physiology. (p. 23)

According to these ideas, the differences between more complex and less complex behavioral mechanisms may lie in the number, subtlety, and lability of the neural connections involved, rather than in the fundamental unit and mode of analysis. Along these lines, for example, the physiologist Bayliss (1920) speculated:

The difference between spinal reflexes and those in which the higher centers, and especially the cerebral cortex, take part is the regularity of the former and the ease with which the latter are modified or abolished by events in other parts of the central nervous system. (p. 508)

Brain and behavior researchers have long believed that it is possible to explain behavioral responses by the application of relatively simple principles. Therefore, the challenge to the modern neurobiologist has been to synthesize and to prove a correct set of hypotheses (or "models") clearly showing the neural mechanism for a mammalian behavior pattern. Using the clear thinking of reflex physiology has been demanded simply by the requirement for deterministic thinking in the absence of clearly stated alternatives. Thus, with the strategies of reflexology and the methods of modern neuroanatomy, neurophysiology, and endocrinology, we have been systematically studying the neural mechansisms for a female mammalian reproductive behavior pattern—lordosis.

C.   Why Lordosis Behavior

1.   Hormones and Reproductive Behavior

Working with a hormone-controlled behavior pattern gives the experimenter a set of powerful manipulations, based on a natural determinant of the behavior, which he can use to study the neural mechanism. Using the tools of experimental endocrinology, he can remove the natural source of the hormone (for instance, by ovariectomy), replace the hormone systemically by injection or other means, implant it locally in specific regions of brain tissue, study the distribution of radioactively labeled hormones by autoradiographic or biochemical means, determine the neurophysiological and neurochemical effects of the hormones, and so forth.

Mating behavior has obvious biological importance. Rodents, such as rats and hamsters, are easily available, and their reproductive behavior is easily elicited in the laboratory in what appears to be a natural form. Adult rats are large enough for detailed electrophysiological and neurochemical analysis. A history of excellent work on the reproductive behavior of rodents and its hormonal control by Beach, Young, Goy, and their collaborators and many other experimentalists further opens the door for a detailed study of neural circuitry.

2.   Lordosis Behavior

Among rodents, lordosis behavior by the female is essential for fertilization to occur, and it is under strong hormonal control by estrogens and progesterone (Beach, 1948; Young, 1961). The amount and intensity of lordosis behavior increase with higher estrogen doses (Table 1-1). Ovariectomized female rats may show lordosis responses after estrogen treatment alone, but they usually show better responses with estrogen treatment followed by progesterone. The same females that respond best

Table 1-1. Lordosis quotient (LQ) and percentage response (PR) of ovariectomized female rats to mounts by male 6 hours after progesterone, following various doses of estrogen priming (mean ± SE; n = 11)

| | Estradiol benzoate priming dose (μg/rat) | | | | | | |
	0	1	3	5	10	20	10×7
LQ	0 ±0	10.8 ±5.4	36.0 ±8.6	68.6 ±11.4	80.6 ±8.5	86.0 ±8.1	95.7 ±1.6
PR (%)	0	45	82	91	91	100	100

From Kow & Pfaff 1975a.

to estrogen alone also tend to respond best to combined estrogen–progesterone treatment (Figure 1–1; Pfaff, 1970b). The actions of these steriod sex hormones on lordosis behavior are not necessarily routed through the pituitary gland, because normal behavioral effects of estrogen and progesterone can be obtained in hypophysectomized female rats (Pfaff, 1970a). Much of the neural analysis reviewed in this book treats the action of estrogen on female reproductive behavior because of the strength and specificity of estrogen-binding phenomena in nerve

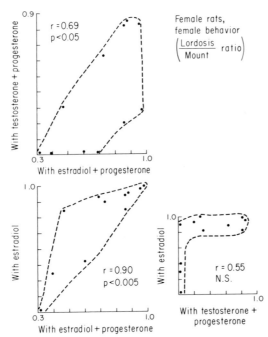

Figure 1–1. Ovariectomized female rats respond to adequate steroid hormone treatment with lordosis behavior. There is a high correlation, across females, in lordosis response frequency with estradiol alone compared to that with estradiol plus progesterone. (From Pfaff, 1970b)

cells, the specificity of its physiological actions, and its action as the primary hormone (both in time and in importance) for facilitating lordosis. Nevertheless, progesterone has an impressive facilitating effect on lordosis in estrogen-primed females, and a theory of its neural mode of action has been presented (Kow, Malsbury, and Pfaff 1974b).

Lordosis behavior has proved to be stereotyped enough (see Section D) for detailed work on its neural mechanisms. Stimuli for triggering it can be determined, its stimulus–response relations are reliable, and its motor topography is simple enough.

For all of these reasons lordosis behavior of the female rodent has proved to be an attractive subject for detailed neuroanatomical and neurophysiological analysis.

The study of the neural circuitry of lordosis behavior is guided by at least two ideas. First, the investigator can follow the routes of determining influences from their first points of contact with the nervous system to the sites of their behavior-determining interaction. For lordosis, as for any other behavior, we have had to find the precise sensory determinants of the behavior (Chapter 2) and to follow relevant sensory signals over the normal neuroanatomical routes using anatomical and physiological techniques (Chapter 3–5). Taking advantage of the hormone dependence of female reproductive behavior, we have studied the binding of steroid sex hormones in brain tissue (Chapter 6). This naturally leads to a study of hypothalamic mechanisms (Chapter 7) and hypothalamic outflow (Chapter 8), which culminate in their impact upon midbrain mechanisms (Chapter 9).

A second guideline is to trace neural mechanisms from regions of relative anatomical simplicity toward more complex neural regions. In the sensory side of the study, this is accomplished simply by following the stimulus information into the central nervous system. For the motor side, we must define the characteristics of the motor response and the muscles involved and use this information to study the relevant motoneurons (Chapter 11). In turn, the actions of descending pathways (including those which carry the hormone-dependent information that originated in the hypothalamus) on the relevant motoneurons can be studied (Chapter 10). In the successful case, systematically gathered neural and behavioral information of this sort should lead to perspectives and laws of the neural basis for behavior (Chapter 12) as well as to a satisfactory paradigm or model for lordosis behavior itself (Chapter 13).

D. Behavioral Description of Lordosis

In a typical case, at the end of a locomotor sequence, including a "hopping and darting" form of locomotion, the estrous female rat comes to an abrupt halt, usually assuming a crouching posture. The male rat, mounting from the rear, first contacts the female's flank region bilaterally with his forearms and the middorsum of her back with his nose and chin. Sometimes his arms touch the anterior border of the female's rear legs. Immediately after the male's forearms touch the female, his four paws grasp further ventrally on her flanks and being palpating (performing rapidly alternating movements on) the skin there. While holding onto her flanks, the male takes at least one step forward with each rear foot, usually achieving a postion such that parts of his lower abdomen and pelvic region are pressing on the skin dorsal and lateral to the female's tailbase (her rump and tailbase region). In some instances his rear legs or feet can be seen contacting the posterior surface of her hips or rear feet. Thus, initial stimuli from the male, before he begins pelvic thrusts, are on the skin of the flank, midback, rump, and tailbase region of the female rat. These stimuli are primarily on the dorsal or lateral surfaces of her body (Pfaff and Lewis, 1974).

After first contact, but before pelvic thrusting by the male, the female's body rocks forward, usually accompanied by a forward extension of both front legs. The rear legs can often be seen to extend or abduct partially. Then, even before pelvic thrusting begins, the first elevation of the rump by the female can sometimes be seen, identified by the fact that the female lifts her perineal skin region off the cage floor surface (Pfaff and Lewis, 1974). In a small number of cases the very beginning of head elevation by the female rat also is seen at about this time.

The male rat typically then begins to thrust his pelvic region rapidly against the rear end of the female. Interthrust intervals are between 40 and 80 milliseconds (Table 1-2; Pfaff, Montgomery, and Lewis, 1977). Only rarely is the initial thrust right into the vagina. More often, the penis contacts the female skin slightly posterior or lateral to the vagina.

Table 1-2. Intervals between visible stimuli from male rat pelvis or forepaws on skin of female rat

Angle of film view	Duration (imsec) (mean ± SD)	Corresponding mean frequency (per sec)
Thrust by pelvis		
Side	63 ± 19	15.9
Ventral	65 ± 21	15.4
Palpation by forepaws		
Side	74 ± 18	13.5
Ventral	84 ± 25	11.9

Note. This is based on a frame-by-frame analysis of film taken at 54 frames per second.

From Pfaff et al., 1977.

During these initial pelvic thrusts, the female extends her rear legs and raises her rump and tailbase region. If the mating encounter is to end in an intromission, subsequent thrusts of the penis contact the vaginal opening and then achieve penile insertion. By the time this deep pelvic thrust, which results in intromission, begins, the female is in the *lordosis posture:* the perineum is elevated, all four legs are extended from the initial crouch position, and the head is elevated. It is obvious that rump elevation by the female during initial penile thrusting is necessary: during the intromittory pelvic thrust by the male, his hindquarters are bent beneath the perineal region of the female such that, in films taken from a ventral view, the back of his body obscures the view of her genital region. Directly after intromission, the male rapidly withdraws the pelvis as he dismounts with a backward springing movement, leaving the female in the lordosis posture: vertebral column dorsiflexed, with the head, rump, and tailbase raised and the thorax lowered (Pfaff and Lewis, 1974).

This narrative description is based on the analysis of films taken from a side view and from a ventral view. Pictures taken from single frames of films of the mating sequence have been presented elsewhere (see Figure 2 in Pfaff et al., 1972).

Average latencies of behavior elements which were easily observable and for which precise times of onset could be determined are given in Table 1-3. Figure 1–2A shows a lordosis in which rump elevation occurred abruptly, beginning less than 200 milliseconds after the forepaws of the male grasped the female's flanks. Initial rump elevation just preceded initial pelvic thrusting, and near-maximal elevation was obtained during extravaginal pelvic thrusting. Figure 1–2B illustrates a

Table 1-3. Mean latencies of behaviors, from time male's paws first grasp female's flanks

Behavior	Latency (msec) (mean ± SE)
Male	
Head touches female's back	12 ± 2[a]
Start of deepest pelvic thrust	399 ± 23
Deepest point of deepest pelvic thrust	587 ± 27
Releases female (paws lifted off flanks)	839 ± 71
Female	
Start of rump elevation	161 ± 11
Start of head elevation	260 ± 15
Point of maximum head elevation	714 ± 48

Note. Time that male's paws first grasp female's flanks is defined as 0 second and latencies are calculated from that point. $N = 85$ mating encounters (mounts), all including intromission.

[a]In some encounters, male's head touches female's back just before paws touch flanks.

From Pfaff & Lewis, 1974.

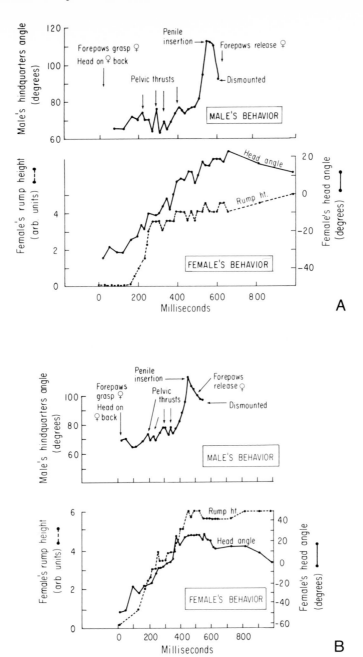

Figure 1–2. Measurements of three individual lordoses. All are graphed in the same way. In measurements of female rat head angle, 0° is horizontal and head elevation is a change toward more positive numbers. In male rat hindquarters angle measurements, 90° is vertical and a forward thrust is shown by a change toward higher numbers. All data are from frame-by-frame analyses of movie films taken from the side view. (From Pfaff & Lewis, 1974)

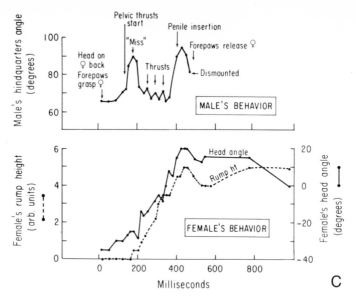

Figure 1–2. (Continued)

similar encounter, except that rump elevation began somewhat earlier, about 100 milliseconds after the forepaws of the male grasped the female's flanks. Rump elevation was also much more gradual, continuing during intitial pelvic thrusting and not reaching maximal height until the intromittory deep pelvic thrust. In this encounter the female's head was raised maximally before penile insertion. Figure 1–2C shows an encounter in which the initial thrust by the male was vigorous but far off to the side from the vagina, apparently constituting a "miss." Subsequent shallow pelvic thrusts by the male were followed by penile insertion. Initial rump elevation and significant increases in the angle of the female's head occurred during and after the miss and continued during shallow pelvic thrusting by the male.

In conventional film analyses, hair, skin, fat, and other tissues reduce the precision with which the skeletal movements that constitute the physical basis for the behavioral response can be followed. With X-ray films, individual bone movements can be visualized, and this information can be used to infer which muscle groups are acting during the behavioral response. We used X-ray cinematography to document skeletal movements during the onset and maintenance of lordosis in the female rat (Pfaff, Diakow, Montgomery, and Jenkins, 1978).

X-ray cinematography confirms the impression that assumption of the lordotic posture by the female rat includes a large change in the angle between the vertebral column at sacral levels and horizontal, and also shows that this vertebral movement is accompanied by a small decrease in the angle between the spine and the innominate, a sizable decrease in the angle between the innominate and the femur, and an increase in the angle between the femur and the crus. Drawings of individual X-ray frames illustrate this change from a nonlordotic (Figure 1–3A) to a lordotic (Figure 1–3B) posture. Following the angles measured as a function of time (Figure 1–4), one can see a rapid decrease in the angle between the vertebral column and horizontal after contact by the male rat. This decrease is accompanied by small, variable changes in the spinal–innominate angle, a rapid decrease in the innominate–femoral angle, and small but quite consistent increases in the angle between the femur and the crus, at the knee (Figure 1–4).

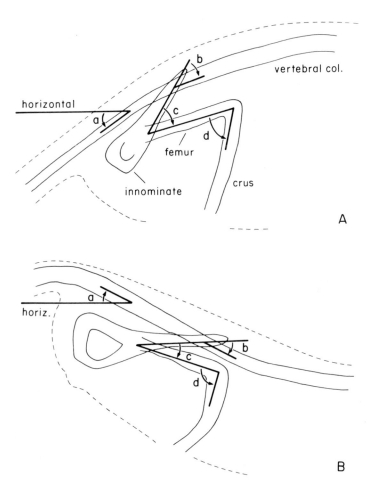

Figure 1–3. Drawings of single frames of X-ray movies taken from the right side of the female rat. The following angles were measured routinely: *a,* horizontal–spinal; *b,* spinal–innominate; *c,* innominate–femoral; *d,* femoral–crural. (A) Female not in lordosis. (B) Female in lordosis. (From Pfaff et al., 1978)

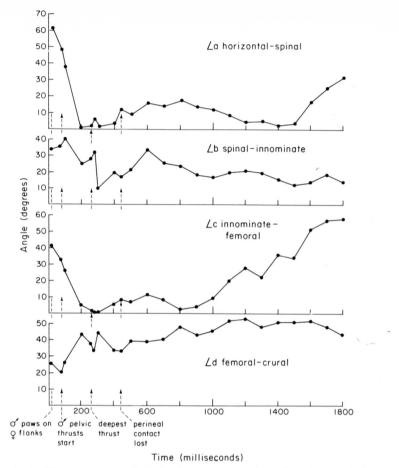

Figure 1–4. Measurements of skeletal movements in a female rat during a representative mating encounter. Changes in bone angles are graphed from before lordosis (time of first contact by male's paws), through the onset and maintenance of lordosis, until female begins to resume locomotion (first movement of female's rear paw). (From Pfaff et al., 1978)

The largest and most consistent average change measured during the onset of lordosis was the change in angle between the vertebral column itself and horizontal (mean change, 59.3°). The decrease in the innominate–femoral angle averaged almost 40°, and the increase in angle at the knee averaged slightly more than 10°. Across encounters, the magnitude of the decrease in the innominate–femoral angle was significantly correlated with the magnitude of the vertebral column change with respect to horizontal ($r = .47$; $p < .05$). Neither the spinal–innominate nor the femoral–crural angle change was significantly correlated with the change in the angle of the vertebral column with respect to horizontal.

Three of the changes in angles (horizontal–spinal, innominate–femoral, and femoral–crural) occurred quite rapidly, beginning between 100 and 200 milliseconds following first contact of the male's paws with the female's flanks (Pfaff et al., 1978).

Forces available to produce the rump and tailbase elevation of lordosis behavior are those acting on the vertebral column itself or those that result from extension of the rear legs. Three arguments from the X-ray cinematography data show that the main lordotic movement must be due to muscles acting on the vertebral column itself. First, as measured in these X-ray observations, the movements associated with the rear legs cannot explain the lordotic rump elevation. The change in the spinal–innominate angle was negligible. The decrease in the innominate–femoral angle was in the wrong direction to explain lordosis. The extension around the knee (increase in the femoral–crural angle) was in the right direction but was too small to account for the large change in the angle of the spinal column with respect to horizontal. Since these leg angle changes cannot explain the large vertebral column movement, and since movements around the ankle mechanically cannot account for the large vertebral column movement, muscles acting on the spinal column itself must be primarily responsible. Second, the only leg angle changing in the right direction to help explain lordosis (increased femoral–crural angle) was not correlated across encounters with the lordotic change in angle between the spinal column and horizontal. Third, even if leg movements would help to account for some portion of rump elevation, they cannot be responsible for the most posterior rump and tailbase, which would droop if only leg action were involved.

Even though the rump of the female usually starts down about the time that perineal contact with the male is lost, the vertebral dorsiflexion of lordosis is usually held some time after that. This finding from the X-ray data simply confirms the common behavioral observation that highly receptive female rats may "hold" the lordotic posture following dismount by the male. Another example of this effect seen in the X-ray films was that the female did not resume locomotion until after all other events in the mating encounter had been finished. These observations show that rump elevation in lordosis cannot be simply a passive result of forces due to pelvic thrusting by the male; an important aspect of the posture must result from muscle action in the female.

In a description of lordosis as a sequence of individual reflexes (Pfaff et al., 1972), based not only on film analyses and X-ray cinematography, but also on experimental analyses of the sensory control of lordosis (see Chapter 2), the male stimulates first the flank and back of the female (with his paws and head), then the region of the tailbase and groin (with his pelvic region), the perineal area, the outer vaginal lip, and finally the deep intravaginal epithelium (during intromission). The female rat extends her legs and raises her tailbase in response to flank stimuli combined with stimuli from the male's first impact in the tailbase and groin area. This response, in turn, allows the male's thrusting pelvis

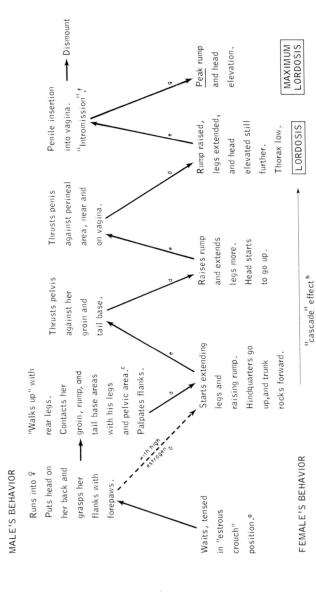

Figure 1–5. Lordosis behavior as a sequence of reflexes in the female rat matched to corresponding responses by the male. (From Pfaff et al., 1972)

greater access to the groin and perineal area, thus intensifying the cutaneous stimulation, which subsequently causes the female to raise her hindquarters further. When she has raised her rump high enough for the male to bend his pelvis underneath, he can exert pressure upward by thrusting on the perineal area. This achieves the stimulation which is sufficient to maximize the lordosis reflex (overall vertebral dorsiflexion) in the receptive female rat (Figure 1–5).

In this description, two main concepts stand out. First, the female's reflex responses to stimuli early in the sequence allow the male to apply subsequent stimuli which are necessary for her subsequent responses. Thus, lordosis behavior can be seen as a sequence of reflexes programmed in the female to match adaptively a corresponding sequence programmed in the male. This "cascade" of reflexes can function as a reproductive isolating mechanism, helping to ensure that only conspecifics endocrinologically competent to reproduce can finish the mating behavior sequence. Second, the female's lordosis reflex is a prerequisite for intromission by the male, rather than the reverse. The number of stages in the reflex sequence (Figure 1–5) has been portrayed as large enough to illustrate recognizable events discretely. Further analysis may identify a larger number of reflex steps. Nevertheless, the combination of film observations, X-ray data, and experimental analyses of sensory control (Chapter 2) presently available prove that successful mating depends on matched series of reflexes in the male and female rat (Pfaff et al., 1972).

Part 1

Triggering the Behavior: Sensory and Ascending Pathways

Chapter 2
Stimulus

A. Stimuli Applied by the Male

During mating encounters that will result in lordosis, the male rat presents olfactory, visual, auditory, and somatosensory stimuli to the female. Gustation is not involved, since the female is not regularly seen to lick the male. Since olfactory, visual, and auditory stimuli are not necessary for lordosis to occur (see Section B), the description below focuses on the somatosensory stimuli.

The parts of the body of female rats contacted by the male in mating encounters which lead to lordosis were mapped by coating the males with a dye just before they were allowed to mount receptive females (Pfaff et al., 1977). The dye was transferred by contact to the hair and skin of the female, providing a visible record of the locations touched by the male. The parts of the female rat's body stained by the dye (i.e., contacted by the male) in a typical case are shown in Figure 2–1.

After mounts with intromissions by the male, accompanied by lordosis in the female, dye was found bilaterally on the flanks (just in front of the rear legs on the side of the body wall), rump (posterior, dorsal, and dorsolateral surface of the body, dorsal to the lateral surface of the rear legs), and tailbase regions. On the ventral surface of the female's body, a dense deposit of dye was always found at the vaginal opening and in the immediate perivaginal region. This deposit was usually much more intense than that in more lateral perineal regions, where dye could be found on the hair (Pfaff et al., 1977).

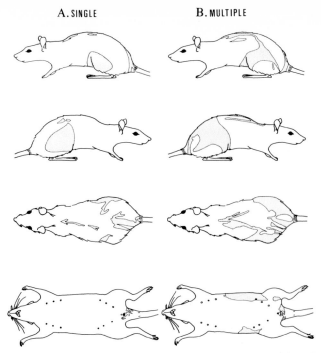

Figure 2–1. Location of dye on hair and skin (stippled areas) of female rat in an individual representative female–male pair after mounts by dye-coated male. (A) After a single intromission. (B) After three additional mounts, one with thrust and two with intromissions. (From Pfaff et al., 1977)

B.   Stimuli Necessary for Lordosis

1.   Noncutaneous Stimuli Are Not Necessary

Female rats that had been surgically deafened, blinded, and rendered anosmic (all three operations were performed on the same rats) displayed strong lordosis reflexes in a high proportion of mounts by the male rat and also responded with lordosis to manual stimulation (Kow and Pfaff, 1976). Indeed, surgical elimination of audition, vision, and olfaction, all in thbe same individual female rats did not have any obvious effect on the display of lordosis. Since gustation is not involved, it appears that sensory input other than somatosensory stimuli is not necessary for lordosis; in other words, somatosensory input alone is sufficient stimulation for triggering the reflex.

In the deafened, blinded, and anosmic females, cutaneous denervation of the flanks, rump, and perineum caused a large decrease in lordosis quotient and abolished the lordosis response to manual stimulation (Kow and Pfaff, 1976). Thus, further analyses of necessary sensory input focused on cutaneous stimuli.

2.   Cutaneous Stimuli

The somatosensory stimuli *necessary* for lordosis can be discovered by selectively reducing those stimuli provided by the male rat or by controlled manual stimulation and observing any decrease in lordosis performance.

Cutaneous denervation of the posterior rump, tailbase, and perineum (Kow and Pfaff, 1976) caused a 51% decrease in the frequency of lordosis in response to mounts by the male rat and a 60% decrease in the lordosis score in manual stimulation tests (Figure 2–2A). Administration of local anesthesia (procaine) to the skin of the posterior rump, tailbase, and perineum (Kow and Pfaff, 1976) replicated the effects of surgical denervation in different female rats and led to the same conclusions regarding the stimuli contributing to lordosis.

When the denervated area of the rump and flanks was enlarged to include the skin on the anterior surface of the rear legs and just in front of the rear legs the lordosis quotient decreased by 80% (Figure 2–2B). Extension of the flank and back denervation even further anterior (Figure 2–2C) did not proportionally increase the magnitude of the effect on lordosis. Extensive cutaneous denervation on the dorsal side of the body, including the rump, flanks, and back, with the perineum remaining untouched, reduced the lordosis quotient by 55% and abolished lordosis responses to manual stimulation (Figure 2–2D). On the other hand, extensively denervation of the ventral side of the body, including the perineum, the inner surface of the legs, and the ventral flank region (where the male's paws palpate the female's skin), virtually abolished lordosis responses both to the male rat and to manual stimulation (Figure 2–2E).

Considering all of these denervation results, it appeared that the most crucial skin areas for lordosis control include the perineum, the tailbase, the most posterior rump, and the most ventral part of the flanks. Denervation of just those skin regions (Figure 2–2F) virtually abolished the performance of lordosis. This pattern of denervation appeared to be optimal for showing cutaneous stimuli necessary for lordosis: a large decrement in lordosis was obtained with a relatively small area of skin desensitized. As an operative control, denervation of the dorsal aspect of the thorax had no significant effect on lordosis.

Vaginal stimulation of the female by the male rat *follows* rump elevation by the female (Pfaff and Lewis, 1974). Furthermore, lordosis can be elicited manually by controlled stimulation by an experimenter, without stimulating the vagina (female rats, Pfaff et al., 1977; female hamsters, Kow, Malsbury, and Pfaff, 1976; female guinea pigs, Young, Dempsey, Hagquist, and Boling, 1937). In fact, lordosis can be observed in female rats in which the vagina has been anesthetized (Bermant and Westbrook, 1966) or removed (Ball, 1934; Kaufman, 1953), or in which vaginal penetration has been prevented by sewing the vagina closed

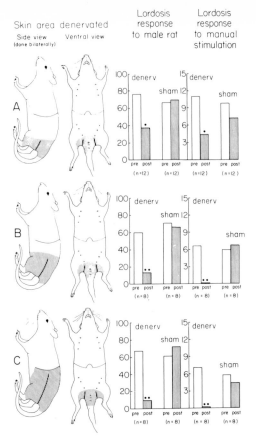

Figure 2–2. Effects of surgical cutaneous denervations of different regions of the female rat's skin on the lordosis reflex. Lordosis was measured in response to mounting by the male rat (lordosis quotient, 0–100) and to manual stimulation by the experimenter (0–15). *Shading:* the area of the female's skin in which all visible cutaneous nerves were cut and the fascia interrupted. *Dark lines* (in the areas of operation): sites of incisions. All operations were bilaterally symmetrical. Graphs show mean lordosis responses before (*pre*) and after (*post*) either denervation or sham operations. Statistical comparisons of postoperative to preoperative results are shown when $n = 6$ or larger: *, $p < .01$; **, $p < .004$. (From Kow & Pfaff, 1976)

(Hard and Larsson, 1968), vaginal masking (Hardy and Debold, 1971), or anesthetizing the male's penis (Kow and Pfaff, 1976). All of these facts point to the conclusion that stimulation of the vagina is not necessary for initiating lordosis.

Since lordosis behavior is greatly reduced or abolished as a result of cutaneous desensitization, it must be concluded that the noncutaneous stimuli still present are not sufficient for triggering the behavior. Similarly, in mating encounters observed during film analyses (Pfaff and Lewis,

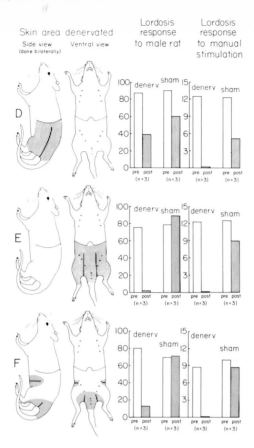

Figure 2–2. (Continued)

1974), no lordoses were ever displayed by female rats before the male had made cutaneous contact—demonstrating the necessity of cutaneous stimuli and the nonsufficiency of noncutaneous stimuli.

In summary, among the regions subjected to somatosensory stimulation by the male rat, the posterior rump, tailbase, and perineum are the most important for lordosis. The small skin region whose desensitization most effectively extended the decrease in lordosis produced by perineum–tailbase–posterior rump denervation was the vertical band of skin on the lateral aspect of the flank and abdomen (touched by the male rat's forearms and forepaws during palpation). Since cutaneous manipulations (surgical denervation and local anesthesia) caused very large reductions in the performance of lordosis, skin receptors themselves must be crucial for lordosis, and, conversely, deep receptors (particularly those in and between muscles) are not sufficient for the normal occurrence of this behavior. All these considerations lead us to the conclusion that cutaneous mechanoreceptors in the hairy skin on the posterior rump, tailbase, and perineum (with additional input from the ventral flanks) play a crucial role in triggering the lordosis reflex in the female rat.

C.   Stimuli Sufficient for Lordosis

The male rat applies natural stimuli as a constellation, so that observation of his behavior alone is not analytical enough to demonstrate the minimal sufficient stimulation. Imitations of the stimuli he applies must be administered separately and in combinations (Diakow, Pfaff, and Komisaruk, 1973; Pfaff et al., 1972) in order to see, under controlled conditions, which somatosensory inputs are sufficient to trigger lordosis. The experimenter applied somatosensory stimuli to the female skin locations contacted by the male rat (Pfaff et al., 1977). Application of light hair-deflecting stimuli bilaterally to the flanks of the female rat did not yield lordosis responses (Figure 2–3A). Neither did light hair-deflecting stim-

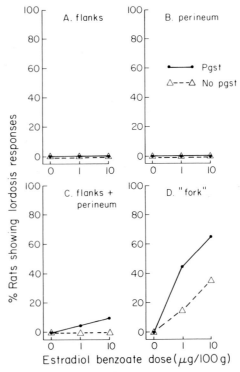

Figure 2–3. Percentage of female rats showing lordosis responses to light cutaneous stimulation. "*Fork*" stimulus consisted of stimulation of flanks followed by pressure on posterior rump, tailbase, and perineum. *Pgst:* progesterone. (From Pfaff et al., 1977)

ulation of the perineum (Figure 2–3B). Light stimulation of the flanks and perineum simultaneously produced lordosis only in a small proportion of females treated with the highest estradiol benzoate dose supplemented by progesterone (Figure 2–3C). In the usual case the minimally adequate cutaneous stimulation was the "fork" stimulus, involving flank stimulation followed by pressure on the posterior rump, tailbase, and perineum (Figure 2–3D). Here, estradiol significantly facilitated the appearance of the reflex response, and progesterone after estrogen treatment had a significant synergistic effect.

It was characteristic of the "fork" stimulation, adequate for producing lordosis, that pressure was exerted upward against the perineum by the experimenter's fingers, and counterpressure was exerted downward against the dorsal surface of the rump by the experimenter's palm. The pressure and counterpressure so exerted were in the direction of "bending the female" toward the lordosis posture. The order of stimulus application was also important for eliciting lordosis. Flank stimulation had to precede (or at least accompany) stimulation of the rump and perineum. Optimally, stimulation of the rump and tailbase is followed quickly by perineal pressure. Usually neither flank nor perineal pressure individually triggered lordosis; for maximal responsivity they must be applied as a set in the proper order. Finally, it was noted informally (Pfaff et al., 1977) that lordosis responsiveness was facilitated by rapid changes in pressure during the application of "fork" stimulation. Gradual applications of pressure were often less effective than fast fluctuations of pressure for eliciting lordosis.

To increase the precision with which physical parameters (place, time, and pressure) of cutaneous stimuli adequate for triggering lordosis are defined, we used pressure sensors to monitor cutaneous stimulation (Kow, Montgomery, and Pfaff, 1979). In turn, the quantitative definition of the adequate stimulus can be used to characterize the effects of estrogen treatment (and other physiological manipulations) and eventually can be used as a key in tracing reflex-relevant activity into and through the central nervous system (see Chapters 3–5).

Airpuffs and brushing, which caused hair movement, were totally ineffective in triggering lordosis (Table 2–1). In the same skin areas, light touch or pressure were effective. Thus, inputs from hair receptors alone, even in skin locations proved (as above) to be crucial for lordosis, are not sufficient for triggering the reflex. During proper stimulation with increasing pressure, lordosis was evoked before the threshold for pain was reached; during ineffective pressure applications, increases in stimulation until signs of pain were observed still did not elicit the reflex. These observations suggest that inputs from high-threshold pressure receptors (or nociceptors) are neither necessary nor sufficient for triggering lordosis.

Light touch or pressure on the skin of the flank, tailbase, and perineum was most effective for triggering lordosis; stimuli on other skin regions

Table 2-1. Effectiveness of different types and locations of mechanostimulation on female rat's skin

Mechanostimulation		No. of rats tested	Percent of rats showing lordosis reflex
Stimulus type	Location(s) stimulated		
Air puffs	Tb + R + P[a]	28	0
Brushing	Tb + R + P[a]	28	0
Light touch (<18 mbar)	DT,F,Tb,R, or P	25	0
	F + P	25	0
	F + Tb	28	7
	Tb + P	25	28
	F + Tb + P	28	68
Pressure (<800 mbar)	DT + F	25	0
	F + Ab	28	0
	F + Tb	29	86
	Tb + P	25	72
	F + Tb + P	29	100

Note. Ab, abdomen; DT, dorsal thorax; F, flank; P, perineum; R, rump; Tb, tail base. One millibar = 1×10^3 dyne/cm^2 = 0.75 mm Hg.

[a]During these stimuli flanks were touched lightly.

From Kow et al., 1979.

or on only one of these three regions were ineffective (Table 2-1). The effective skin regions are those contacted by the male during mating (Pfaff et al., 1977) and shown by cutaneous denervation to be essential for lordosis (Kow and Pfaff, 1976). They are also effective for triggering lordosis in hamsters (see below). Within the effective skin regions the percentage of the rats showed lordosis depended on the total area stimulated. Light touch applied to flanks, tailbase, and perineum was more effective than that on only flanks plus tailbase, tailbase plus perineum, or flanks plus perineum. Also, light touch on flanks, tailbase or perineum alone was never effective (Table 2-1). Similarly, the three-location pressure stimulation was more effective than any of the two-location stimuli. Thus, in rats, as in hamsters (Kow et al., 1976), inputs from mechanoreceptors at different locations can be summated to trigger lordosis.

Such a spatial summation is illustrated further by the measurement of pressure required for lordosis. Figure 2–4 shows that the three-location stimulation not only caused a higher percentage of females to show lordosis, but also required less pressure than the two-location stimulation. Thus, sensory input from flanks, tailbase, and perineum can summate to help trigger lordosis; for a given effectiveness, an increase in the area of stimulation lowers the pressure required (Kow et al., 1979).

For a given pressure, higher estrogen doses induced more animals to respond with lordosis (Figure 2–5). For a given level of lordosis performance, increases in estrogen dose lowered the pressure required. From

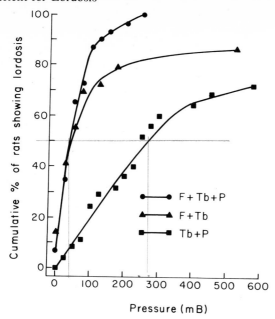

Figure 2–4. Cumulative percentage of rats showing lordosis as a function of pressure applied. Skin regions stimulated were flanks (*F*), tailbase (*Tb*), and perineum (*P*). Pressures were measured from the tailbase in *F* + *Tb* stimulation and from the perineum in the other two types of stimulation. (From Kow et al., 1979)

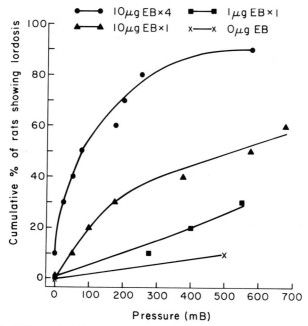

Figure 2–5. Effect of different doses of estradiol benzoate (*EB*) on the effectiveness of pressure stimulation of the flanks, tailbase, and perineum for eliciting lordosis reflex. (From Kow et al., 1979)

this observation and the work summarized above we conclude that, within effective locations on the skin of a female rat, lordosis performance can be increased by increasing any of three factors: stimulus pressure, total area stimulated, and the amount of estrogen (Kow et al., 1979).

In order to see if the quantitative results of these analytical experiments on sufficient stimuli were in the same range as those produced during natural mating, we measured the pressure on the skin of the female rat during natural mating with male rats (Kow et al., 1979). Indeed, the range of stimulus pressures (Table 2–2) applied by the male rats were comparable to that used in manual stimuli effective for triggering lordoses, indicating that the more analytical, artificially produced stimuli can substitute for those produced by the male in physiological experiments. The peak amounts of pressure applied by the male differed according to whether or not the males thrusted (Table 2-2). In simple mounts, pressures applied were lower and lordoses were less strong and frequent. Within categories of behaviors by the males, greater pressures were associated with stronger lordoses (Kow et al., 1979). When stimuli from the male were divided into blocks according to pressure on the female's skin (Figure 2–6), it became evident that greater pressure leads to a higher probability of triggering lordosis and higher lordosis reflex strength.

Lordosis is triggered in female hamsters by stimuli on the same skin areas as in rats (Kow et al., 1976; Pfaff et al., 1972). The mean ratings of lordosis responses to standard cutaneous stimulation in each zone of the body are presented for female and male hamsters in Figure 2–7. Stimulation of Zones I and II of the head region always disrupted lordosis in both females and males. Stimulation of an area between the front

Table 2-2. Pressure applied to female's tailbase by male rats during mating encounters

Male's behavior	Strength of lordosis evoked	No. of rats	Pressure[a] (mbar)	
			Mean ± SE	Range
Simple mount	None	13	84 ± 10	27–136
	Weak	2	104 ± 35	69–139
Mount with thrusts	None	64	145 ± 7	43–325
	Weak	87	175 ± 8	48–427
	Strong	41	238 ± 14	48–432
Intromission	None	5	87 ± 19	32–139
	Weak	19	186 ± 11	96–277
	Strong	23	202 ± 20	75–448
Ejaculation	Strong	6	192 ± 15	144–240

[a]Pressure used is highest pressure recorded in each mating encounter before male's deep pelvic thrust.

From Kow et al., 1979.

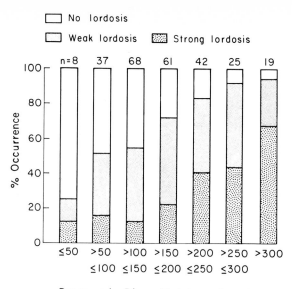

Figure 2–6. Occurrence and strength of lordosis reflex as a function of the pressure applied by male rats during mating behavior. (From Kow et al., 1979)

shoulder and the last rib was relatively neutral. Stimulation became more effective for eliciting lordosis in both female and male hamsters when applied to the part of the skin posterior to the last ribs. Within this area of skin, cutaneous stimulation on every zone elicited lordosis in all female and in some male hamsters, and never caused disruption of lordosis. Ranking the skin zones in terms of mean lordosis rating revealed that the relative sensitivities of the zones were almost identical for the

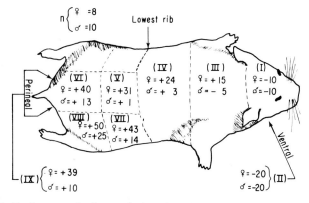

Figure 2–7. Body map of a hamster showing division into nine testing zones and the average rating of lordosis responses to cutaneous stimulation in each zone. *Plus sign:* elicitation of lordosis, the larger the number, the better the average quality of lordosis. *Minus sign:* disruption of lordosis. (From Kow et al., 1976)

two sexes (r = .98). Upon stimulation of zones where lordosis could be elicited, the mean lordosis rating was higher in female than in male hamsters (Kow et al., 1976).

Thus, as in rats, sufficient sensory information for eliciting lordosis in female hamsters is provided by the flanks, rump, and perineum. However, whereas rats require rather strong stimulation on all three skin areas, weak stimuli on any one of them can trigger lordosis in female hamsters.

D. Summary

Cutaneous stimulation on the flanks of female rats, followed by pressure on the posterior rump, tailbase, and perineum (a) is applied by the male rat during mating, (b) is necessary for lordosis, and (c) is sufficient for lordosis.

Chapter 3
Primary Sensory Neurons

A. Distribution of Peripheral Sensory Nerves

In the female rat, sensory nerves supplying the perineal skin region (input from which is crucial for lordosis) run with the pudendal nerve (Kow and Pfaff, 1973). The receptive field of the primary sensory branch of the pudendal nerve occupies an area of ipsilateral skin: its medial boundary is approximately on the midline; its maximum longitudinal extent is from the level of the lowest nipple to about the midpoint between vagina and anus; and its lateral boundary is between the abdomen–thigh junction and the heel (Figure 3–1). In fact, for most of the perineal skin, there is no sensory supply from other nerves (Kow and Pfaff, 1975b). During dorsal root recording experiments, electrophysiological responses to cutaneous stimulation in the perineal region were measured before and after the pudendal nerve was severed. As expected, before the nerve was severed handsome responses to cutaneous perineal stimulation were recorded from dorsal root L_6 (Figure 3–2A). After the pudendal nerve was severed, the response to perineal stimulation disappeared completely (Figure 3-2B). The disappearance of the response was not due to cutaneous receptor damage, for the response could still be recorded on the peripheral section of the cut pudendal nerve. Thus, over the main portion of the receptive field of the pudendal nerve, covering most of the perineal region, there is no sensory supply from other nerves.

Electrical recording from the pudendal nerve revealed an orderly pattern of cutaneous sensitivity in the perineal region (Kow and Pfaff, 1973). At a series of points on a grid across the pudendal nerve receptive field, we measured thresholds (milligrams of force) for pudendal nerve response. The most sensitive points were regularly in the middle of the receptive field (Figure 3–3). Moreover, median response thresholds were correlated, across preparations, to overall receptive field size. Median

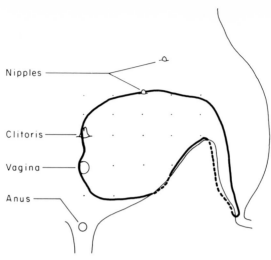

Nipples

Clitoris

Vagina

Anus

Figure 3–1. Location of receptive field of the perineofemoral branch of the pudendal nerve in a representative estrogen-treated female rat. *Thick line:* the receptive field, determined by recording nerve responses during stimulation of the skin with a small camel hair brush. *Broken line:* the field extending slightly beyond the ventral surface. (From Kow & Pfaff, 1973)

thresholds from preparations with large receptive fields were lower than those from preparations with small receptive fields (Figure 3-3). Notably, the lowest threshold points in all preparations covered the areas of skin contacted by the preliminary thrusting of the male rat during mating encounters.

Input from other skin regions on the female rat important for lordos-

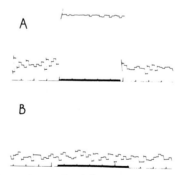

A

B

Figure 3–2. Effect of severing pudendal nerve on dorsal root multiunit responses: recordings of dorsal root L_6. (A) Before pudendal nerve was severed. (B) After pudendal nerve was severed. *Thickened portions of time marker lines:* skin within the pudendal nerve receptive field was brushed. The dorsal root response to skin stimulation occurred before (A) but not after (B) the pudendal nerve was cut. (From Kow & Pfaff, 1975b)

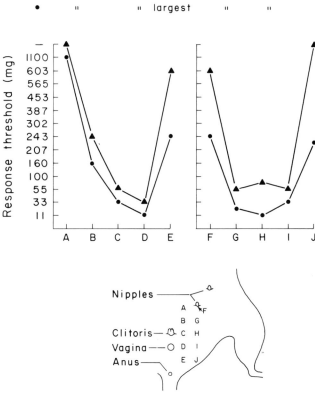

Figure 3–3. Differences between thresholds across preparations according to receptive field size. *A–J* (on the abscissa): grid points whose positions are shown in the drawing on the bottom. Preparations with large receptive fields tend to have lower thresholds for phasic nerve response than those with small receptive fields. (From Kow & Pfaff, 1973)

is—the ventral flanks and posterior rump—is carried via peripheral nerves which are not as well characterized as the pudendal nerve. However, from dorsal root recording experiments (Kow and Pfaff, 1975b) we have deduced some general features of the routes followed by these sensory nerves. For instance, incisions that completely circumscribed a skin area stimulated in the female rat did not eliminate dorsal root electrical responses to that stimulation (Figure 3–4). Thus, an important sustaining sensory nerve supply must come from directly below the skin area stimulated. When an incision was made (Figure 3–5A) and just the skin area stimulated was undercut, the dorsal root electrophysiological response was still not eliminated (Figure 3–5B). Separation of the skin from the underlying tissues did not eliminate the dorsal root response to

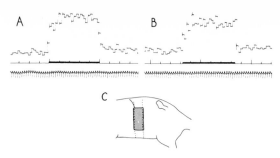

Figure 3–4 A–C. Results of a "curcumscribing incision" experiment. (A) Polygraph record of the multiunit response of dorsal root T_{12} to the brushing of the skin area (shown in panel C) before the circumscribing incision of the skin. *Bottom trace:* Electrocardiogram. (B) After the incision. (C) Area of skin (*shaded*) stimulated by brushing. *Dotted lines:* borders of T_{12} receptive field. *Solid line:* path of the circumscribing incision. (From Kow & Pfaff, 1975b)

skin stimulation on the flanks of the female rat until the undercut area was much larger than the area stimulated (Figure 3–5C). From the results of both the "circumscribing incision" experiments (Figure 3–4) and the "skin undercutting" experiments (Figure 3–5), we conclude that the sensory nerve supply to an area of skin (for example, on the flanks of

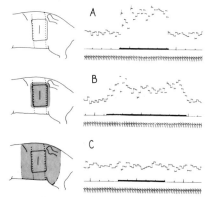

Figure 3–5 A–C. Results of a "skin undercutting" experiment. Drawings on the left indicate the conditions under which the corresponding recordings on the right were made. *Dotted lines:* borders of the L_1 receptive field. *Solid rectangular line:* skin area brushed during each recording. *Vertical line inside enclosed rectangle:* incision made in order to undercut the skin. *Shading:* extent of the undercut. Tracings on the right show polygraph records of dorsal root L_1 multiunit responses to the brushing (*thickened time marker line*) of the indicated skin area under the following conditions: (A) With central incision but not undercut. (B) With small undercut, (C) With large undercut. Only the large undercut abolished the dorsal root response. *Bottom trace:* electrocardiogram. (From Kow & Pfaff, 1975b)

the female rat) comes not only from directly underneath that skin but also from surrounding areas of skin (Kow and Pfaff, 1975b).

B.   Sensory Neuron Types

We recorded single unit activity from primary sensory neurons using micropipettes inserted into the dorsal root ganglion (Kow and Pfaff, 1979). We chose dorsal root ganglion L_6 in female rats because this spinal level receives input from the perineal skin (Kow and Pfaff, 1975b), which is crucial for the triggering of lordosis. The neurons were divided into categories based on their responses to the stimuli used, including lordosis-relevant stimulation (Table 3–1). Cutaneous mechanoreceptive units constituted 84% of the recorded population. None of these neurons showed resting discharge; responses never outlasted stimulation.

Hair units were those that responded to hair movement but showed no sustained responses to stimulation with the von Frey hair or pressure stimulation. For example, some units responded to the movement of down (D) hairs —fine wavy hairs that grow in groups out of individual follicle openings. Others responded to the movement of guard (G) hairs — distinctly larger than down hairs, and straight, with one hair per follicle opening. Each hair unit responded to the movement of only one type of hair. Therefore, each unit was simply named according to the type of hair that evoked its response (Table 3-1).

Units that responded to hair movements but also showed sustained responses to skin deformation were categorized as *hair–skin* units (Table 3-1). Among the hair–skin units, Tylotrich hair–Haarscheibe (Type I) units (Figure 3–6) responded to the movement of a Tylotrich hair and to von Frey hair stimulation of the cutaneous dome (Haarscheibe, tactile pad, Type I receptor) with which the Tylotrich hair was associated. Typically, such a unit initially responded with a high firing rate, which then decreased to a sustained lower rate. The Haarscheibe is very sensitive to deformation, but with a threshold von Frey hair a unit response could be evoked only from the elevated dome, not from the flat skin surrounding it.

Skin deformation units were those that responded to von Frey hair or pressure stimulation, but not to hair movement (Table 3-1). Fourteen of these units responded to the von Frey hair, but not to pressure stimulation. Since these neurons responded to the deformation of small spots on the skin, they were named punctate skin deformation (PSD) units.

Other skin deformation units, probably the most important for lordosis, responded not only to the deformation of small spots of skin, but also to pressure on areas of skin. These were called *pressure units* (Figure 3–7). Pressure units started to fire when the pressure applied reached a

Table 3-1. Number of units and response profiles for each unit type recorded in rat L⁷ dorsal root ganglion

Type of unit	No. of units	Percent of units responding to each form of stimulation						
		Hair movement (hair type)	Air puff	Brushing	von Frey hair On– off	von Frey hair Sustained	Pressure	Movement of tail or leg
Cutaneous mechanoreceptive units								
Hair								
G hair	57	100 (G only)	47	100	44	0	0	0
D hair	47	100 (D only)	77	100	47	0	0	0
C hair	29	100 (C only)	55	100	62	0	0	0
T hair	3	100 (T only)	33	100	33	0	0	0
Unidentified hair	18	100	39	100	50	0	0	0
Hair–skin								
Type I	37	100 (Ty only)	8	97	3	97	95	0
L hair	4	100 (L only)	0	100	0	75	75	0
Bimodal	6	100	17	100	17	83	33	0
Skin deformation								
Punctuate skin deformation	14	0	0	29	7	93	0	0
Pressure	48	0	0	8	6	94	100	0
Noncutaneous units								
Muscle–joint	19	0	0	0	0	0	0	100
Deep pressure	1	0	0	0	0	0	100	0
Unresponsive units	29	0	0	0	0	0	0	0

From Kow & Pfaff, 1979.

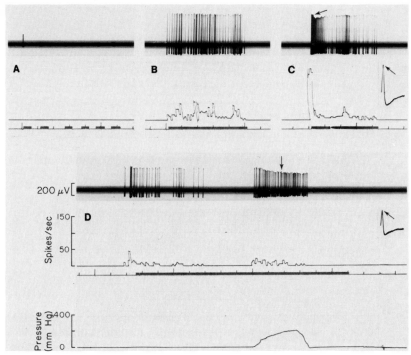

Figure 3–6 A–D. Responses of a type I unit to different forms of stimulation. Each time division denotes 1 second. (A) Airpuffs, (B) Brushing, (C) Von Frey hair, (D) Pressure. A response was evoked by mere contact with the pressure sensor, and then by the small amount of pressure at the very beginning of pressure application. Despite reductions in spike amplitude during responses the shape of the potential remained the same, as shown by the inserts in panels C and D (taken from the spike trains as indicated by *arrows*). (From Kow & Pfaff, 1979)

threshold level that was different for different units. Beyond the threshold, increasing pressure caused the firing rate to increase.

C. Quantitative Features of Responses

1. Thresholds

The mean threshold for responses by pressure units was 131 mbar (Kow and Pfaff, 1979). This is within the range of cutaneous pressure effective for evoking lordosis behavior (Chapter 2).

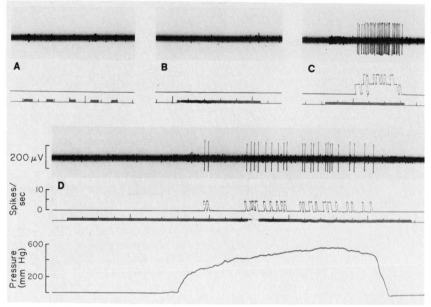

Figure 3-7. Responses of a pressure unit. Figure arrangement and conventions as for Figure 3-6. In response to pressure (panel D), the firing rate was correlated with stimulus intensity, with a threshold of about 400 mm Hg. (From Kow & Pfaff, 1979)

2. Receptive Fields

Receptive fields for skin deformation units were small, averaging 0.97 mm² (Kow and Pfaff, 1979). This is much smaller than the area of skin which needs to be contacted in order to evoke lordosis behavior (Chapter 2). Therefore, summation of input from different units must be required for lordosis to occur.

3. Time Course

When a von Frey hair is applied to the skin, two types of responses may be evoked: phasic and tonic (Kow and Pfaff, 1973). In the phasic response, neural activity is evoked only at the onset and the end of application of the von Frey hair to the skin. Tonic responses are, with few exceptions, superimposed on the phasic "on–off" response. Tonic responses (also called "slow adapting" or "sustained" responses) are maintained throughout the period of stimulus application. Estrogen effects on receptive field size and response thresholds were apparent in measurements of phasic responses, but not tonic responses (Kow and Pfaff, 1973).

D.   Effect of Estrogen

During recording from the pudendal nerve (Kow and Pfaff, 1973) we measured receptive field size in estrogen-treated and untreated ovariectomized female rats. The mean receptive field size of the pudendal nerve in estrogen-treated females (175.6 mm^2) was 22% larger ($p < .001$) than in the untreated ovariectomized females (144.4 mm^2). While estrogen had a significant effect, there also was a considerable overlap in the ranges of individual receptive field sizes between the estrogen-treated and control groups. One aspect of the receptive field expansion in the estrogen-treated rats was that the probability of extension of the receptive field laterally onto the leg was significantly higher in the estrogen-treated than in the untreated group. The increase in receptive field size caused by estrogen was also found in the same experiments (Kow and Pfaff, 1973) by an independent line of evidence: the difference between estrogen-treated and untreated rats in the percentage of preparations responding to von Frey hair stimulation at each point of a grid superimposed on the pudendal nerve receptive field. In both estrogen-treated and untreated females, the percentage of preparations responding was 100% at grid points in the center of the pudendal nerve receptive field. Toward the boundaries of the receptive field, the average percentages of preparations responding declined, and at these grid points estrogen-treated rats were significantly more responsive than untreated rats. The estrogen effects appeared only for phasic responses. There were no reliable differences between groups in the tonic responses of the pudendal nerve to steady stimulation.

At each point of the grid (superimposed on the pudendal nerve receptive field) the threshold (in milligrams) for response was measured with von Frey hairs both for phasic and tonic responses (Kow and Pfaff, 1973). For phasic responses, we found a trend for the estrogen-treated rats to have a lower threshold than the untreated group. Of the 17 grid points at which median thresholds were obtained, the estrogen-treated rats had lower thresholds at 14 points, equal at 1 point, and higher at only 2 points ($p < .005$). This trend also appeared to be specific for phasic responses, because there were no reliable differences in thresholds for tonic responses between estrogen-treated and untreated rats.

Thus, the estrogen effect is appropriate to the type of stimulation applied by the male rat during normal induction of lordosis behavior. Rapid pelvic thrusting by the male, contacting the female's skin in the pudendal nerve receptive field, certainly results in phasic responses, which we find to be estrogen sensitive, rather than tonic responses, which are not estrogen sensitive (Kow and Pfaff, 1973). Nevertheless, in these pudendal nerve recordings, there was considerable overlapping between estrogen-treated and untreated groups, both in receptive field size and sensitivity. In the overall behavioral responses of these animals there was no overlapping: all estrogen-treated animals showed strong lordoses, while none of the untreated control group did. Therefore, unless specific, strongly estrogen-sensitive receptors were masked by our stimulation and recording methods, the peripheral somatosensory estrogen effect we discovered could not by itself account for the overall estrogen effect upon the lordosis reflex.

The conclusion that estrogen can increase the receptive field size of the pudendal nerve in ovariectomized female rats was also reached independently by Komisaruk, Adler, and Hutchison (1972). In determining the receptive field size of the entire pudendal nerve, they also found that estrogen treatment can cause a statistically significant expansion in the median receptive field size. In agreement with our results, their data also showed a large range of individual receptive field sizes within each group, causing considerable overlap between groups and indicating that the estrogen effect as presently measured has not been an all-or-none phenomenon.

In later experiments (Kow and Pfaff, 1979) we measured the size of the receptive field for the entire L_6 dorsal root. It was significantly larger in estrogen-treated female rats than in control untreated ovariectomized females. However, in these experiments, comparisons of data from single unit recording showed that, although receptive field sizes tended to be larger in the estrogen-treated than in the control rats, there were no statistically significant differences for any individual unit type between the two groups. Similarly, for individual single units, thresholds for response were not significantly different between the estrogen-treated and control groups. Thus, it appears that the observation of a statistically significant primary sensory estrogen effect depends on the large effective sample achieved in whole-nerve recording or whole–dorsal root receptive field measurements.

E.   Which Cells Trigger Lordosis?

1.   Cutaneous Receptors Involved: A Process of Elimination

Lordosis is triggered reliably by specific forms of cutaneous mechanostimulation. Therefore, the units found in peripheral nerves and the dorsal root ganglion (Kow and Pfaff, 1979) which do not respond to cutaneous mechanical stimulation are irrelevant for triggering lordosis. Likewise, noncutaneous units, such as muscle–joint units, cannot be responsible for evoking this behavior.

Cutaneous mechanical stimuli that just deflect hairs, such as brushing on the skin and airpuffs, never evoked lordosis (Chapter 2). All types of hair units in the dorsal root ganglion responded to brushing and many responded to airpuffs (Kow and Pfaff, 1979). Therefore, activation of hair units could not be sufficient for lordosis behavior. Slowly increasing pressure on the skin could trigger lordosis (Kow et al., 1979). Hair units either did not respond to the stimulation or they responded only briefly at its beginning, and not during the behaviorally relevant pressure increase. Therefore, their activation could not be necessary for the behavior to occur. Possibly, during stimulation from the male rat involving a high frequency of pelvic thrusting, hair units could have some role. The input from hair units at about the same time as input from other more important units might summate to increase the overall effectiveness of stimulation from the male rat. However, during controlled manual stimulation, sensory information from hair units does not seem to contribute to triggering lordosis.

Hair–skin units (such as Type I units) responded to brushing (which does not evoke lordosis), indicating that their activation is not sufficient for triggering lordosis behavior. Moreover, although Type I units responded to pressure, their pressure threshold was extremely low—lower than the pressures needed to trigger lordosis in a majority of rats. Again, their activation cannot be sufficient for the reflex. Nevertheless, the temporal patterns of response by Type I units to pressure might be discriminated centrally, in the cord, and have some behavioral significance. Furthermore, whereas input from Type I units themselves may not be sufficient, their sustained responses to pressure stimuli might summate with input from other types of receptors and strengthen the behavioral output.

A relatively large area of the female rat's skin is contacted during pressure leading to lordosis. Punctate skin deformation units do not respond to such pressure (Kow and Pfaff, 1979); therefore, activation of these units is not necessary for the triggering of lordosis. During stimuli from the male rat, local skin deformation may play a greater role, but it is clear that lordosis behavior can occur without activity in punctate skin deformation units.

The only remaining unit type is the pressure-responsive unit. These units did not respond to airpuffs or brushing on the skin—stimuli that did not lead to lordosis. Pressure units did respond to the type of pressure stimulation that does evoke lordosis. Indeed, the range of pressure thresholds for units of this type was comparable to the range for triggering lordosis responses (see Figure 4-4).

We conclude that the pressure units are the most important type of dorsal root ganglion single units for triggering lordosis behavior. Their stimulus requirements for firing most closely fit the pattern of stimulus requirements for lordosis behavior as a whole. Although stimulation from the male rat mounting, for instance, might cause a barrage of action potentials from most of the dorsal root ganglion cutaneous-responsive unit types, pressure units are the best individual candidates for controlling the behavioral response.

These analyses, based on primary sensory neuron single unit recording, are consistent with and extend hypotheses derived from cutaneous denervation experiments (Kow and Pfaff, 1976). Based on the stimulus requirements for the behavior as a whole (Chapter 2) and the nature of the sensory neuron types discovered, we can proceed to consider which pressure-responsive cutaneous receptor types might or might not be involved. For example, receptors such as Pacinian corpuscles—which have optimal stimulating frequencies of 100–400/second and are very difficult to stimulate at frequencies below 40/second (Burgess and Perl, 1973)—are unlikely to be crucial for lordosis. The predominant frequencies of repetitive stimuli by the male rat are below 20/second (Pfaff et al., 1977). Another type of pressure-responsive cutaneous receptor to be eliminated is that associated with C-fibers, which requires strong stimulation for at least 150 milliseconds (Burgess and Perl, 1973). Information from these receptors, though signaling pressure, would not arrive quickly enough to account for lordosis behavior, which has an average latency of 161 milliseconds (Pfaff and Lewis, 1974).

The type of pressure units whose stimulus requirements fit those for lordosis behavior as a whole are likely to receive their input from the same types of cutaneous receptors as the Type II units previously described in cats (Burgess, Petit, and Warren, 1968; Iggo, 1966). Like Type II units, the rat's pressure units were slowly adapting, were not associated with tactile domes, and had small receptive fields. They gave sustained responses to punctate deformation of the skin and were sensitive to pressure exerted over a larger area. If the pressure-sensitive units we found in female rats are the same as Type II units, then they are likely to be associated with Ruffini endings (Burgess and Perl, 1973).

Thus, if any single chain of sensory events plays a crucial role in triggering the lordosis response, it appears that pressure on the L_6 receptive field of female rats deforms Ruffini endings, leading to an activation of Type II fibers (pressure units), which yields an input to the spinal cord effective in eliciting lordosis.

2.   Requirements for Summation

Since the receptive fields of skin deformation units are much smaller than the skin areas that must be stimulated to evoke lordosis, it must be that inputs from pressure units are summated to generate the behavioral response. In addition, it may be that, even for a given skin area, inputs from less effective types of cutaneous receptors (for instance, Type I units or hair units) are summated with inputs from pressure receptors to facilitate the behavior. Another example of summation is that flank stimulation, ineffective in triggering lordosis by itself, strengthens the response to rump and perineal pressure. (Behavioral evidence for summation was reviewed in Chapter 2.)

Similarly, stimuli can be summated to facilitate lordosis in female hamsters. The percentage of hamsters displaying lordosis increases steadily when larger areas of the skin are stimulated (Kow et al., 1976; Manogue, Kow, and Pfaff, 1980a). Light bilateral cutaneous stimulation triggers significantly stronger lordosis responses than unilateral stimulation (Manogue, et al., 1980a). Moreover, although visual, olfactory, and auditory stimuli by themselves are neither sufficient nor necessary to elicit lordosis in female hamsters, information from them can summate with somatosensory input to evoke reproductive behavior (Manogue et al., 1980a; Murphy, 1974; Noble, 1973).

F.   Summary

Stimulation from mounting by the male rat, which leads to lordosis, would cause a barrage of action potentials from most of the cutaneous mechanoreceptive unit types in the dorsal root ganglion. However, among all primary sensory neurons, only pressure units and Type I units gave sustained responses to a lordosis-triggering type of pressure stimulation. Stimulus requirements for the pressure units most closely fit the pattern of stimulus requirements for lordosis behavior as a whole. In order to evoke lordosis, summation across pressure units certainly occurs, and summation with other unit types may also be involved. If any single chain of events has the central role, however, it is that pressure on the crucial skin areas deforms Ruffini endings, thereby activating (Type II) pressure units.

Chapter 4
Spinal Interneurons

A. Distribution of Sensory Input

Somatosensory input was followed from the skin to the dorsal roots by recording electrical responses of each of the dorsal roots from thoracic level 11 (T_{11}) through sacral level 3 (S_3) (Kow and Pfaff, 1975b). Altogether, the receptive field of dorsal roots T_{11} through S_1 covers the skin of the dorsal and lateral sides of the body from just anterior of the last rib to the end of the fur on the tail, including the rear limbs and perineal skin (Figure 4–1). An important area for the control of lordosis, the skin of the flanks contacted by the forepaws and forearms of the male rat is mapped onto dorsal roots L_1 and L_2. Crucial for lordosis, the skin of the posterior rump, perineum, and tailbase give input to dorsal roots L_5, L_6, and S_1 (Figure 4–2). Thus, during mating behavior which leads to lordosis, sensory input to spinal interneurons comes primarily over dorsal roots L_1, L_2, L_5, L_6, and S_1. In the rat, dorsal roots L_1 and L_2, carrying input from the skin of the flanks, end in the cord at vertebral levels T_{12} and anterior T_{13}. Dorsal roots L_5, L_6, and S_1, bringing input from the posterior rump, perineum, and tailbase, end in the cord at vertebral level L_1 (Kow and Pfaff, 1975b).

Fibers from the posterior trunk of the body traveling over dorsal root L_5 go preferentially to the lateral side of the dorsal horn. Those traveling over dorsal roots L_6 and S_1 from the dorsal and lateral trunk skin also go to the lateral side of the spinal gray matter, while those with input from the perineum tend to favor the medial side of the dorsal horn. We deduced this from spinal single unit recording in which units were classified according to whether they were found in the medial or lateral half of the spinal gray matter (Kow, Zemlan, and Pfaff, 1980a). Each unit's location in the spinal cord was then related to the location of its receptive field on the skin (Table 4–1). Spinal units with receptive fields on the distal or ventral portion of a dermatome tend to be located in the

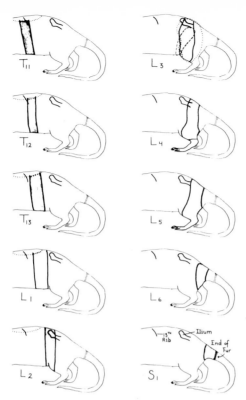

Figure 4–1. Representative locations of cutaneous receptive fields (*shaded areas*) for dorsal roots T_{11} through S_1 in the rat. *Dotted line* (in T_{11} through L_2): extent of the separation of skin from the underlying tissues due to the dorsal approach to the cord for electrode insertion. For L_3, the largest (*dotted line*) and smallest (*dashed line*) examples of receptive field size are superimposed on the representative field (*shaded area*). The 13th rib is the most posterior rib. The crest of the ilium is indicated. (From Kow & Pfaff, 1975b)

medial half of the spinal gray, while units with receptive fields on the proximal or dorsal parts of a dermatome tended to be located in the lateral half of the spinal gray (Table 4–1). Excitingly, Mendell, Sassoon, and Wall (1977) found that in cats, lumbar spinal units that are sensitive to "long-distance" effects from skin far anterior to their normal receptive fields—i.e., to input from the flanks—are located preferentially on the lateral side of the dorsal horn. Thus, in female rats, those units on the lateral side of the dorsal horn which receive input on the posterior trunk (posterior rump and tailbase) from initial pelvic thrusts by the male (crucially related to the triggering of lordosis) may be the same units that are sensitive to long-distance input from flank skin, which facilitates lordosis.

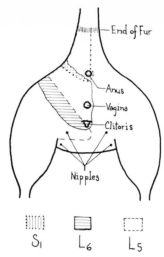

Figure 4–2. Portion of the cutaneous receptive fields of dorsal roots L_5, L_6, and S_1 viewed from behind the rat with the tail elevated. (From Kow & Pfaff, 1975b)

B.   Unit Types Defined by Sensory Input

1.   Types Found

By means of micropipettes, extracellular recordings were made of the single unit activity of 345 spinal units in segments L_5, L_6, and S_1 (dorsal root level) in urethane-anesthetized female rats. In order to analyze sensory mechanisms for triggering lordosis, we studied unit responses to skin pressure which evokes lordosis and many other mechanical cutaneous stimuli (Kow et al., 1980a).

Among units *not* relevant for lordosis, hair movement units responded to movement of individual hairs, airpuffs, and brushing (hair units) or required the simultaneous movement of many hairs (field units) (Table 4–2). Subdermal units responded only to the manipulation of muscles or joints or to pressure on tissues beneath the skin. Other units showed no response to the routine stimuli used, including lordosis-relevant skin pressure, but might show responses to pain, vaginal probing, or no stimuli at all.

Type I units showed sustained responses to the identation of tactile domes, possibly contributing to lordosis. They were very sensitive to pressure. Mere contact of the pressure sensor with the receptive field, without any appreciable pressure, could evoke a long-lasting response in these units.

Skin deformation units in the spinal gray were essentially pressure-sensitive units. They showed sustained responses to pressure on skin not associated with tactile domes (Figure 4–3). Most of them were

Table 4-1. Relationship between mediolateral unit location and receptive field location

Unit location in spinal grey	L_5				L_6-S_1		
	Back	Perineum	Thigh	Leg–Foot	Back	Perineum	Anogenital
Medial	1[a]	7	7	15[a]	3[b]	24[b]	10
Lateral	14[a]	8	6	5[a]	12[b]	11[b]	9

Note. Values indicate number of units with receptive field on part of body indicated.

[a]Back versus leg–foot significantly different ($p < .005$).

[b]Back versus perineum significantly different ($p < .05$).

From Kow et al., 1980b.

Table 4-2. Number of units and response profile for each unit type recorded in rat dorsal root segments L_5, L_6, and S_1

Type of unit	No. of units	Movement of individual hairs	Air puffs		Brushing			Von Frey hair sustained			Pressure			Muscle-Joint (M-J)		
			↑ᵃ	↓ᵇ	↑	→	↑↓ᶜ	↑	→	↑↓	↑	→	↑↓	↑	→	↑↓
Hair movement																
Hair (H)	41	100	71	0	100	0	0	0	0	0	0	0	0	0	0	0
Field (F)	31	0	48	0	97	3	0	0	0	0	0	0	0	0	0	0
Type I	16	94	63	0	94	0	0	100	100	0	100	0	0	0	0	0
Skin deformation																
Pressure→ ↑ (P ↑)ᵃ	44	0	0	0	0	0	0	34	0	0	100	0	0	0	0	0
Pressure→ ↓ (P ↓)ᵇ	7	0	0	0	0	0	0	0	29	0	0	100	0	0	0	0
Pressure→ ↑ or ↓ (P ↑↓)ᶜ	3	0	0	0	0	0	0	0	33	33	0	0	100	0	0	0

Percent of units responding to each form of stimulation

Hair–skin															
H or F + P ↑	51	25	51	6	84	10	6	59	0	0	100	0	0	0	0	0
H or F + P ↓	15	13	33	0	93	7	0	0	13	0	0	100	0	0	0	0
F + P ↑↓	2	0	0	0	0	0	100	0	0	50	0	0	100	0	0	0
Subdermal															
M-J	43	0	0	0	0	0	0	0	0	0	0	0	0	79	0	21
Deep pressure	4	0	0	0	0	0	0	0	0	0	75	25	0	0	0	0
Hair–skin–subdermal															
P ↑ + M-J (+F)	15	0	13	0	33	0	0	40	0	0	100	0	0	60	13	27
P ↓ + M-J (+F)	6	0	17	17	33	17	0	0	17	0	0	100	0	33	17	50
P ↑↓ + M-J (+F)	4	0	0	0	50	0	0	0	0	0	0	0	100	50	0	50
M-J + F	13	0	23	8	92	8	0	0	0	0	0	0	0	39	15	46
Other units	50	0	0	0	0	0	0	0	0	0	0	0	0	0	0	0

[a] ↑, increased firing rate.

[b] ↓, decreased firing rate.

[c] ↑↓, either increased or decreased firing rate depending on location or exact form of stimulation.

From Kow et al., 1980b.

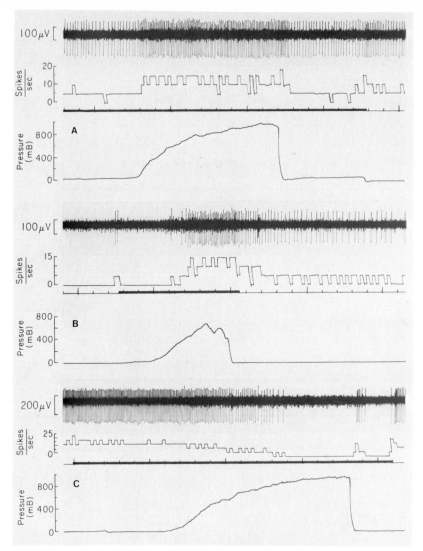

Figure 4–3 A–C. Responses of pressure-sensitive neurons recorded in the spinal cord. (A) Most of these units were excited by pressure on the skin. (B) Some responses outlasted the stimulus. (C) A few units were inhibited by cutaneous pressure. (From Kow et al., 1980b)

excited by pressure (Figure 4–3A, B). When continuously increasing pressure on the receptive field of such units reached a threshold level, their firing rate would increase to a plateau level, which then was maintained despite further increases in pressure. Upon release of pressure, most pressure-sensitive units promptly returned to their resting level of firing (Figure 4–3A). The firing rates of a few remained higher for some time (Figure 4–3B). Finally, a few pressure-sensitive units were inhibited by pressure in ways almost parallel to the ways that the others were excited (Figure 4–3C).

Hair–skin units may also be relevant for lordosis. When subjected to pressure alone, they behaved as pressure-sensitive units in every respect. When give simple hair deflection stimuli, they behaved like hair movement units; when hair movement stimuli and skin deformation were applied simultaneously, more complicated responses appeared.

2.   Locations in Cord

Most of the spinal gray units recorded were in laminae IV–VIII and X, while a few were in laminae I–III or motor nuclei. Hair and Type I units were located almost exclusively in the dorsal horn, usually lamina IV. Field units were found most frequently in lamina V. Units showing excitatory responses to pressure, most relevant for lordosis, had the center of their distribution in the intermediate gray. Units with inhibitory responses to pressure were somewhat more ventral. Finally, units responding only to subdermal stimulation, such as manipulation of muscles and joints, were found most ventrally. Thus, spinal neurons responding to stimulation of structures on the surface of the body (hair) tended to be located more dorsally in the spinal gray, while units evoked from deeper structures tended to be located more ventrally. In further analyses encompassing the full dorsal–ventral extent of the spinal gray, we found that the incidence and firing rate of spontaneously active units were greater for ventral than for dorsally located units (Kow et al., 1980a). Receptive field sizes and (to a limited extent) thresholds were also greater for more ventrally located units.

3.   Comparison to Primary Sensory Units

Compared with single units recorded from the sixth lumbar dorsal root ganglion of female rats (Kow and Pfaff, 1979), units in the spinal gray (Kow et al., 1980a) showed a wider variety of unit types, more complicated responses, much larger receptive fields, and higher resting activity. Although all primary cutaneous units were silent in the resting state, spontaneously active units were found for virtually every unit type in the spinal gray. In fact, the proliferation of new unit types in the spinal gray can be explained simply by two factors: the capacity to show inhibitory responses (following from the presence of spontaneous activity), and the convergence of primary unit types (see Section D.2; Kow et al., 1980a).

C.   Quantitative Features of Neuronal Responses

1.   Thresholds

Pressure thresholds for all pressure-sensitive units were in the range effective (Kow et al., 1979) for triggering lordosis behavior (Figure 4–4). Type I units were by far the most sensitive, while the variety of pressure-responsive spinal unit types sensitive to pressure on skin outside the tactile domes had thresholds ranging from 93 to 272 mbar (Table 4–3). From the comparison of thresholds (Figure 4–4), it seems clear that the easiest way to explain lordosis triggering is that sufficient pressure on the skin excites dorsal root ganglion pressure units, which in turn alter the firing rates (mostly, excite) of pressure-sensitive spinal units in the intermediate gray.

2.   Receptive Fields

Receptive fields of pressure units were confined to the side of the body ipsilateral to the unit's location. They were much smaller than the skin area that must be stimulated to trigger lordosis. For example, receptive fields for units simply excited by pressure ranged roughly from 50 to 200 mm^2 (Kow et al., 1980a). Within various unit types, receptive field sizes for cells located more ventrally were significantly larger than those for cells located more dorsally.

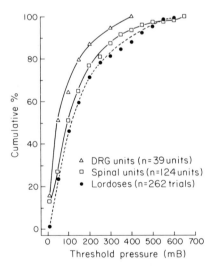

Figure 4–4. Relationship of pressure thresholds for pressure-sensitive neurons in L$_6$ dorsal root ganglion (*DRG*) and spinal cord to threshold for lordosis behavior. (From Kow et al., 1980b)

Table 4-3. *Thresholds (mean ± SE) for pressure-responsive units*

Type of unit[a]	von Frey hair ($\log_{10}$ force in mg)		Pressure (mbar)	
Type I	3.14 ± .22	(7)[b,c]	12 ± 5	(11)[b,c]
P ↑	4.50 ± .15	(9)	183 ± 26	(36)[d]
P ↑ + H or F	4.36 ± .09	(20)	93 ± 13	(35)[d]
P ↑ + M-J (+F)	4.37 ± .12	(5)	198 ± 40	(14)
P ↓	4.56	(1)	135 ± 49	(6)
P ↓ + H or F	4.31	(1)	214 ± 71	(9)
P ↓ + M-J (+F)	4.31	(1)	175 ± 49	(5)
P ↑ ↓ and P ↑ ↓ +				
Excitation	4.56	(1)	252 ± 79	(7)
Inhibition	5.06 ± .13	(2)	272 ± 83	(8)

[a]P, pressure; H, hair; F, field; M-J, muscle or joint; ↑, excitation; ↓, inhibition.

[b]Values in parentheses indicate the number of units.

[c]Significantly lower than all other thresholds ($p < .001$).

[d]Significantly different from each other ($p < .01$).

From Kow et al., 1980b.

D. Implications

1. Which Interneurons Control Lordosis?

Of all the spinal interneurons recorded, pressure-sensitive skin deformation units appeared to be the most relevant for triggering lordosis. They responded to pressure, which is a lordosis-relevant stimulus. They did not respond to the other forms of cutaneous stimulation which are not effective for triggering the reflex. Finally, their pressure thresholds were similar to those for triggering the behavior as a whole. Neurons excited by pressure sustained their response throughout stimulation, and throughout their dynamic range the total number of spikes evoked increased with increasing pressure. All of these neuronal characteristics are well correlated with the behavioral fact that increasing the intensity of pressure applied increases the probability of triggering a lordosis reflex (Kow et al., 1979). Thus, units excited by pressure could serve as interneurons mediating excitatory information that eventually activates motoneurons and the musculature for executing the behavior.

It is easy to rule out certain other types of interneurons. Hair units, field units, muscle–joint units, deep pressure units, nociceptive, vaginal probing and unresponsive units (and combinations of these types)—all of which did not respond to lordosis-relevant cutaneous pressure—could not be essential for the behavior.

Finally, spinal neurons that responded positively to pressure and also to other forms of stimulation may have some role. The response of these units to the multiple types of cutaneous stimulation from the male rat may act to preserve and even increase the lordosis-relevant response. The roles of other types of units—those whose responses to other stimuli were opposite in sign to those for pressure—in lordosis, if any, would have to be complex. Finally, Type I units, which responded to Tylotrich hair movement as well as to tactile dome indentation, responded to pressure at thresholds too low to trigger lordosis behavior. Furthermore, the response evoked by pressure was not proportional to the amount of pressure applied. Thus, while Type I units could contribute to the overall synaptic excitation involved in spinal circuits, they could not be sufficient by themselves to trigger lordosis.

2. Convergence: Feature of Neuronal Responses and Mechanism of Summation

The most striking observation in the comparison of primary and spinal neuronal responses was the evidence for the *convergence* of primary units onto spinal interneurons. During dorsal root ganglion single unit recording (Kow and Pfaff, 1979) hardly any bimodality units were observed, and every identified hair unit or hair–skin unit could be evoked from only one type of hair. In contrast, in the spinal gray (Kow et al., 1980a), many units responding to both hair movement and skin deformation were found, as well as units responding to many other combinations of cutaneous stimulation. Moreover, many hair units could be evoked by more than one type of hair.

Convergence of primary sensory units onto spinal interneurons could also be seen among units of the same modality: receptive field sizes for corresponding types of units increased greatly from primary sensory to spinal neurons (Kow and Pfaff, 1979, compared with Kow et al., 1980a). Even with stimulation methods and protocols held constant across the two recording experiments, the convergence ratios (calculated from average receptive field sizes of spinal units divided by primary units) were 8 for Type I units, 17 for down hair units, 10 for guard hair units, and 61 for pressure units.

Convergence of lordosis-relevant cutaneous stimulation from larger numbers of primary units onto smaller numbers of spinal interneurons is an obvious way in which behavioral summation effects could occur. Examples were given in Chapter 2 (also see, for example, Kow et al., 1979; Pfaff et al., 1977) which showed that stimuli covering smaller areas might not evoke lordosis or might evoke only weak reflexes whereas stimuli over a larger area could evoke a strong reflex. The mechanism of such summation effects could simply be that stimulation of the larger area is sufficient to excite interneurons on which greater amounts of sensory information have converged.

In turn, further convergence of sensory information from the inter-neurons described above must be necessary for a complete behavioral mechanism. The rather large amount of skin area that must be stimulated to trigger lordosis (Kow et al., 1979) exceeds the receptive field areas of the pressure-sensitive neurons described above. Thus, an individual pressure-sensitive unit of the type demonstrated thus far, even if maxi-mally excited, could not be sensitive over a sufficient area to trigger the behavior. Therefore, information evoked in several pressure-responsive interneurons must converge. Motoneurons are candidates for such con-vergence because they can receive inputs from pressure receptors (Egger and Wall, 1971; Engberg, 1964), but higher order spinal interneurons or supraspinal neurons (Kow and Pfaff, 1977) are also possible sites for convergence.

3. Unanswered Questions

Further questions about the spinal interneurons of interest must be answered using electrophysiological and neuroanatomical techniques. Where do the pressure-sensitive spinal interneurons project? Which among them excite or inhibit other spinal interneurons? Do any synapse directly on motoneurons? Do any project to the other side of the spinal cord, fostering the integration of lordosis as a behavior triggered by bilateral stimulation and characterized by bilaterally symmetrical re-sponses?

Functional questions may also be answered by means of electrophys-iological recording. Exactly how does stimulation from the skin of the flanks potentiate responses to pressure on the rump and perineum? Where does the bilateral integration of the reflex take place? At what point do the major estrogen effects enter the spinal circuitry? Likewise, where do the descending influences know to be involved have their major impact?

E. Summary

Primary sensory units responsive to pressure converge on pressure-sensitive interneurons in the intermediate gray of the lumbar spinal cord of female rats to participate in triggering lordosis behavior (Figure 4–5).

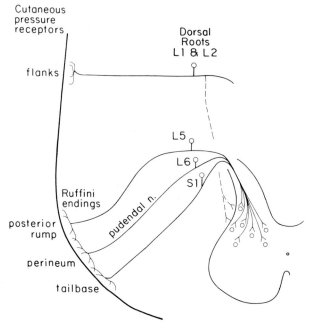

Figure 4–5. Summary of neurons with important roles in the triggering of lordosis behavior by cutaneous stimuli.

Chapter 5
Ascending Neural Pathways

A.   No Lordosis in Spinal Rats

To see whether connections between the spinal cord posterior to thoracic
levels and supraspinal structures are required for lordosis, hormone-
primed female rats were studied before and after complete transection of
the spinal cord at low thoracic levels. All sham-operated rats showed
strong lordosis reflexes before and after surgery. None of the rats
receiving complete spinal transections performed lordosis after surgery,
even in tests done 3 months and more after transection (Kow, Montgomery, and Pfaff, 1977). Even pharmacological attempts to facilitate
lordosis failed to bring out the reflex in spinally transected hormone-
primed female rats (Kow et al., 1980b). Thus, supraspinal control is
required for the normal lordosis reflex. The net effect of this control
must be facilitation of lordosis-relevant circuitry at segmental spinal
levels.

B.   Locations of Critical Pathways

In order to find where critical ascending or descending pathways run in
the spinal columns for the control of lordosis, selective transections of
individual or combinations of spinal columns were performed in hormone-
primed female rats (Kow et al., 1977). Females with bilateral transections
of dorsal columns, dorsolateral columns, or the entire dorsal half of the
spinal cord performed lordosis in a normal way (Table 5–1). Therefore,
no fibers running through the dorsal half of the spinal cord to or from the
brain can be critical for lordosis. Similarly, females with bilateral transections of fibers in the ventromedial columns (even in addition to
transection of dorsal columns or the entire dorsal half of the cord) still
performed lordosis normally. Thus, no fibers other than those in the
anterolateral columns are critical for lordosis (Figure 5–1, top row).

Table 5-1. Average (mean ± SLM) preoperative (Pre) and postoperative (Post) lordosis reflex scores and postoperative performance (POP) in female rats following different transections

Group	n	Type of transection	Manual stimulation test				Lordosis quotient			
			Pre	Post	POP[a]	p	Pre	Post	POP[a]	
Sham	9		7.6 ± .4	8.6 ± .3	114 ± 4	< .01	81 ± 4	94 ± 3	117 ± 3	< .001
Severe Sham	6		7.0 ± .4	7.5 ± .2	108 ± 6	NS	74 ± 5	85 ± 7	117 ± 12	NS
DC	11		7.5 ± .4	7.5 ± .2	102 ± 4	NS	82 ± 5	86 ± 4	108 ± 7	NS
DL	4		7.1 ± .4	8.8 ± .4	124 ± 4	< .01	79 ± 7	85 ± 6	108 ± 2	< .02

DH	12	$7.6 \pm .2$	$8.1 \pm .3$	107 ± 4	NS	81 ± 3	79 ± 4	98 ± 5	NS
M	4	$7.1 \pm .5$	$6.0 \pm .9$	83 ± 12	NS	97 ± 5	88 ± 5	91 ± 4	NS
DH + VM	3	7.2 ± 1.0	$7.7 \pm .2$	111 ± 15	NS	95 ± 5	78 ± 4	83 ± 7	NS
AL Attempts	13	$7.9 \pm .2$	$2.5 \pm .6$	32 ± 8	$< .001$	79 ± 4	47 ± 12	56 ± 14	$< .02$
AL + DL	1	7.0	0	0	—	97	58	60	—
DH + AL	1	7.5	0	0	—	83	0	0	—

[a]POP calculated as (Post/Pre) × 100.

From Kow et al., 1977.

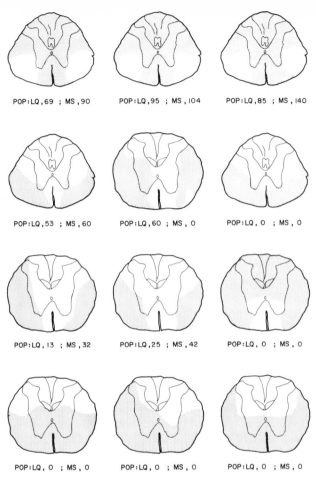

POP:LQ,69 ; MS ,90   POP:LQ,95 ; MS ,104   POP:LQ,85 ; MS ,140

POP:LQ,53 ; MS , 60   POP:LQ,60 ; MS , 0   POP:LQ, 0 ; MS , 0

POP:LQ, 13 ; MS , 32   POP:LQ,25 ; MS ,42   POP:LQ, 0 ; MS , 0

POP:LQ, 0 ; MS , 0   POP:LQ, 0 ; MS , 0   POP:LQ, 0 ; MS , 0

Figure 5–1. Greatest cross-sectional extent of spinal transection (*shaded area*) in 12 female rats. Lordosis reflex results are shown below each drawing: *POP*, postoperative performance, as a percentage of preoperative performance; *LQ*, lordosis quotient, in tests with male rats; *MS*, manual stimulation tests. (From Kow et al., 1977)

Large bilateral transections of the anterolateral columns caused severe losses in the strength and frequency of lordosis behavior (Figure 5–2). Effective transections usually included some ventromedial or dorsolateral column fibers and were accompanied by abnormalities of locomotion.

Fibers necessary and sufficient for lordosis must run in the anterolateral columns. Because large transections are required to eliminate the reflex, these fibers are probably dispersed throughout the anterolateral columns. They may also be involved in (or interspersed with other fibers involved in) other aspects of motor control. Candidate descending systems are the lateral vestibulospinal and lateral reticulospinal tracts (see Chapter 10). The candidate ascending system is the anterolateral system of fibers, whose projections are described below.

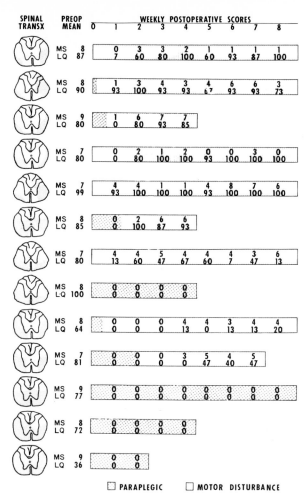

SPINAL TRANSX	PREOP MEAN		WEEKLY POSTOPERATIVE SCORES								
		0	1	2	3	4	5	6	7	8	
MS 8 LQ 87		0 7	3 60	3 80	2 100	1 60	1 93	1 87	1 100		
MS 8 LQ 90		1 93	3 100	4 93	3 93	4 67	6 93	6 93	3 73		
MS 9 LQ 80		1 0	6 80	7 93	7 85						
MS 7 LQ 80		0 0	2 80	1 100	2 100	0 93	0 100	3 100	0 100		
MS 7 LQ 99		4 93	4 100	1 100	1 100	4 93	8 100	7 100	6 100		
MS 8 LQ 85		0 0	2 100	6 87	6 93						
MS 7 LQ 80		4 13	4 60	5 47	4 67	4 60	4 7	3 47	6 13		
MS 8 LQ 100		0 0	0 0	0 0	0 0						
MS 8 LQ 64		0 0	0 0	0 0	4 13	4 0	3 13	4 13	4 20		
MS 7 LQ 81		0 0	0 0	0 0	3 0	5 47	4 40	5 47			
MS 9 LQ 77		0 0	0 0	0 0	0 0	0 0	0 0	0 0	0 0		
MS 8 LQ 72		0 0	0 0	0 0	0 0						
MS 9 LQ 36		0 0	0 0								

☐ PARAPLEGIC   ☐ MOTOR DISTURBANCE

Figure 5–2. Lordosis reflex results for female rats with anterolateral column transections. Greatest cross-sectional extent of each transection (*shaded area*) is shown. Preoperative (averaged) results and postoperative data are shown for each animal: *MS*, manual stimulation tests, top score of 10; *LQ*, lordosis quotient, in tests with male rats, top score of 100. Survival time of each animal after surgery is shown by the length of the bar enclosing the postoperative scores. Large bilateral anterolateral column transections led to decreased lordosis reflex performance. (From Kow et al., 1977)

C.   Projections of Ascending Pathways

We located the cells of origin of axons rising through the anterolateral columns by transecting an anterolateral column and applying horseradish peroxidase (HRP) to the cut fibers (Zemlan, Leonard, Kow, and Pfaff, 1978).

Cell bodies giving rise to long ascending axons in the anterolateral columns are primarily located in the contralateral spinal gray (Figure 5–3). They can be found deep in the dorsal horn, and in the intermediate spinal gray, and some are in Rexed layers VII and VIII. The range of depth covered by these cells corresponds roughly to that covered by pressure-sensitive spinal interneurons described above (Chapter 4).

We studied the projections of axons ascending in the anterolateral columns by transecting anterolateral column fibers and following ascending degenerating axons using the Fink-Heimer technique (Zemlan et al., 1978). Our results add detail to and extend to the rat previously reported findings (Anderson and Berry, 1959; Mehler, 1969; Nauta and Kuypers, 1958).

Fibers ascending from the anterolateral columns maintain their ventrolateral position in the medulla (Figure 5–4). Some axons terminate in the lateral reticular nucleus. Some terminate in the medullary reticular formation, including the ventral reticular nucleus (Figure 5–4J, K) and the nucleus gigantocellularis (Figure 5–4H, I).

A significant number of degenerating fibers leave the ventrolateral medulla and enter the inferior cerebellar peduncle (5–4H). Some of these fibers end in the vestibular complex, while others travel dorsally to the cerebellum.

Further rostral, some fibers from the anterolateral column begin to shift dorsally from the ventrolateral brainstem (Figure 5–4F, G). Some terminate in the reticular formation of the pons. Others eventually sweep dorsally to run near and among fibers of the lateral lemniscus (Figure 5–4E).

At the junction of the pons and mesencephalon, some fibers from the anterolateral column turn medially and terminate in the central gray of the midbrain or diffusely dorsal and lateral of the central gray (in the reticular formation and the intercollicular region) (Figure 5–4C).

The last remaining fibers continue rostrally in the classical spinothalamic tract (Figure 5–4A, B; Zemlan et al., 1978).

Many of these ascending fiber subsystems from the anterolateral column can be ruled out as far as critical lordosis control is concerned. Fibers terminating in the dorsal column nuclei are not involved, since the entire dorsal column system is not relevant for lordosis. Spinocerebellar fibers and fibers terminating in the lateral reticular nucleus (a precerebellar way station) do not participate critically in lordosis control, because essential cerebellar participation has been ruled out for several reasons. Female rats that have undergone massive or total removal of the cerebellum still perform lordosis (Zemlan and Pfaff, 1975). Cerebellar inputs and outputs do not seem to be involved. Massive lesions of the inferior olive and destruction of deep cerebellar nuclei or the superior cerebellar peduncle have had no effect on lordosis (Modianos and Pfaff, 1976b). The spinofacial tract originates only in the cervical cord and ends in a nucleus irrelevant for rear body posture, and hence is not involved in lordosis. Finally, spinothalamic fibers are not important for lordosis,

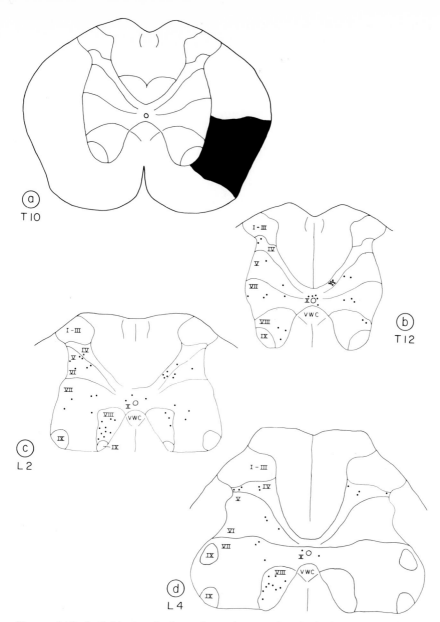

Figure 5–3. Individual spinal cord sections at levels indicated showing the location of labeled cells after transection and HRP application to the severed axons of the right anterolateral column. The number of labeled cells charted is the number per 100-μm section. Abbreviations as in Figure 5–4. (From Zemlan et al., 1978)

since their loss in female cats (Bard, 1939) and female rats (Manogue et al., 1980a) has not led to the loss of female mating reflexes.

The remaining anterolateral column ascending fibers—i.e., spinoreticular axons, spinovestibular fibers, and axons which end in and around the central gray of the midbrain—are candidates for carrying lordosis-relevant sensory information.

D. Responses of Cells in the Brainstem

1. Medulla

Nerve cells in the reticular formation of the medulla may receive lordosis-relevant sensory information (see above) and are good subjects for chronic recording techniques. Thus, we recorded from cells in the

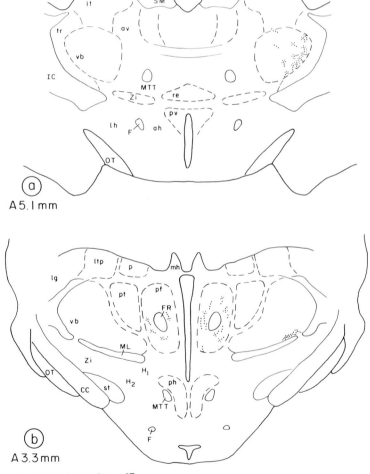

Figure 5–4. See legend, p. 67.

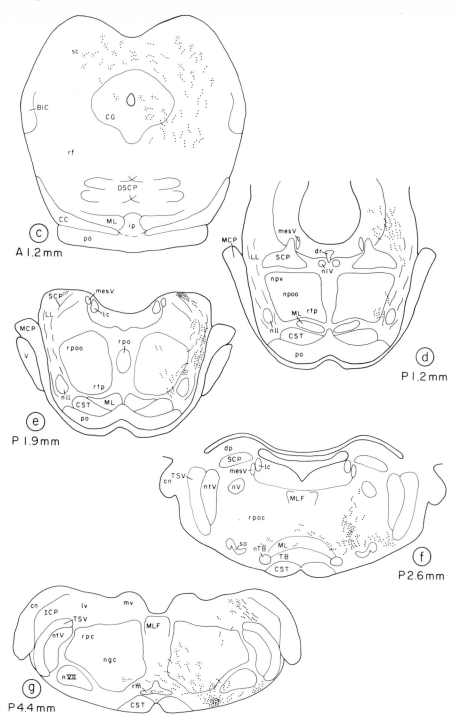

Figure 5–4. (Continued). See legend, p. 67.

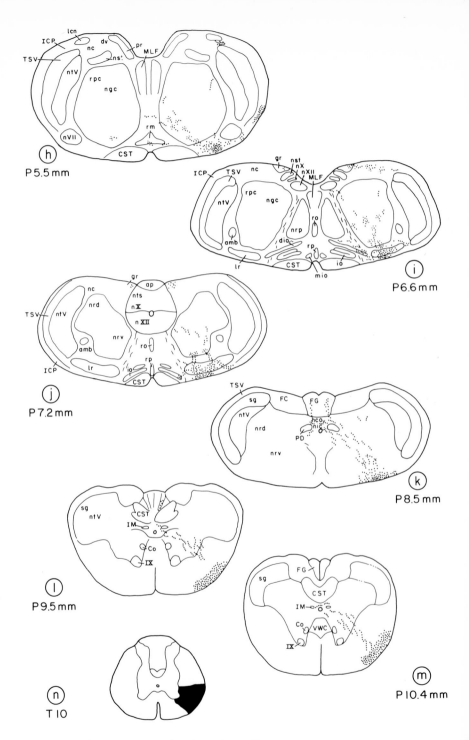

Figure 5-4. (Continued). See legend, p. 67.

Figure 5–4. Degeneration observed after transection of the right anterolateral column at T_{10}. *Coarse dots:* degenerating fibers. *Fine dots:* preterminal degeneration. Stereotaxic coordinates are indicated at the bottom of each brain section. *Numerals on brain sections refer to cranial nerves:* V, trigeminal nerve; *VII,* facial nerve; *VIII,* vestibular nerve; *IX,* glossopharyngeal nerve; *X,* vagus nerve. Numerals on spinal cord sections refer to the cytoarchitectonic layers; *I* through *IX,* laminae I through IX; *X,* substantia grisea centralis. (From Zemlan et al., 1978) *Abbreviations: ah,* anterior hypothalamic nucleus; *amb,* nucleus ambiguus; *ap,* area postrema; *av,* anterior ventral hypothalamic nucleus; *BIC,* brachium of the inferior colliculus; *CC,* crus cerebri; *CG,* central gray matter; *cmg,* central nucleus of the medial geniculate body; *cn,* cochlear nucleus; *CST,* corticospinal tract; *dio,* dorsal inferior olive; *dmnX,* dorsal motor nucleus of the vagus nerve; *dp,* dorsal parabrachial nucleus; *dr,* dorsal raphe; *DSCP,* decussation of the superior cerebellar peduncle; *dv,* descending vestibular nucleus; *F,* fornix; *FC,* fasciculus cuneatus; *FG,* fasciculus gracilis; *gr,* nucleus gracilis: H_1, H_2, fields of Forel; *iC,* interstial nucleus of Cajal; *IC,* internal capsule; *ICP,* inferior cerebellar peduncle; *IM,* nucleus intermediomedialis; *io,* inferior olive; *ip,* interpeduncular nucleus; *lc,* locus ceruleus; *lcn,* lateral cuneate nucleus; *lg,* lateral geniculate body; *lh,* lateral hypothalamic nucleus; *LL,* lateral lemniscus; *lr,* lateral reticular nucleus; *lt,* lateral thalamic nucleus; *ltp,* lateral thalamic nucleus, posterior portion; *lv,* lateral vestibular nucleus; *mb,* mammillary body; *MCP,* middle cerebellar peduncle; *mes V,* mesencephalic nucleus of the trigeminal nerve; *mh,* medial habenular nucleus; *mio,* medial inferior olive; *ML,* medial lemniscus; *MLF,* medial longitudinal fasciculus; *mmg,* marginal nucleus of the medial geniculate body; *MTT,* mammillothalamic tract; *mv,* medial vestibular nucleus; *nc,* cuneate nucleus; *nco,* nucleus commissuralis; *ngc,* nucleus reticularis gigantocellularis; *nic,* nucleus intercalatus; *nll,* nucleus of the lateral lemniscus; *nOT,* nucleus of the optic tract; *npv,* ventral parabrachial nucleus; *nrd,* dorsal reticular nucleus; *nrp,* paramedian reticular nucleus; *nrv,* ventral reticular nucleus; *nst,* nucleus of the solitary tract; *nTB,* nucleus of the trapezoid body; *ntV,* nucleus of the spinal trigeminal tract; *nIV,* nucleus of the trochlear nerve; *nV,* motor nucleus of the trigeminal nerve; *nVII,* nucleus of the facial nerve; *nIX,* dorsal motor nucleus of the glossopharyngeal nerve; *nX,* dorsal motor nucleus of the vagus nerve; *OT,* optic tract; *p,* pretectal nucleus; *PC,* posterior commissure; *PD,* pyramidal decussation; *pf,* nucleus parafascicularis; *ph,* posterior hypothalamic nucleus; *po,* pontine nuclei; *pr,* nucleus prepositus; *pt,* posterior thalamic nucleus: *pv,* paraventricular nucleus; *r,* red nucleus; *re,* nucleus reuniens; *rf,* reticular formation; *rm,* raphe magnus; *ro,* raphe obscurus; *rp,* raphe pallidus, *rpc,* parvocellular reticular nucleus; *rpo,* raphe pontis; *rpoc,* nucleus reticularis pontis caudalis; *rpoo,* nucleus reticularis pontis oralis; *rtp,* pontine tegmental reticular nucleus; *sc,* superior colliculus; *SCP,* superior cerebellar peduncle; *sg,* substantia gelatinosa (Rolandi); *SM,* stria medullaris; *snc,* substantia nigra, zona compacta; *snl,* substantia nigra, lateral portion; *snr,* substantia nigra, reticular portion; *so,* superior olive; *st,* subthalamic nucleus; *ST,* solitary tract; *TB,* trapezoid body; *tr,* reticular thalamic nucleus; *TSV,* spinal trigeminal tract; *vb,* ventrobasal complex; *VWC,* ventral white commissure; *X,* area x, accessory vestibular nucleus; *Z,* area z, accessory vestibular nucleus; *Zi,* zona incerta.

nucleus gigantocellularis in unanesthetized freely moving, hormone-primed female rats (Kow and Pfaff, 1980). Many units responded to cutaneous stimuli on the flanks. However, the effective stimuli were not of the pressure type: the responses were those of the field unit type (responses to hair movement over a rather large area), and the cells responded the same whether lordosis was triggered or not (Figure 5–5). Medullary reticular units have not responded to pressure on the perineum in unanesthetized freely moving animals. The only indications of such a response have come from experiments with anesthetized females. We have not found medullary reticular units whose firing rates are tightly locked in a phasic manner to the occurrence of lordosis. Importantly, medullary reticulospinal units—identified antidromically by electrical stimulation of the spinal cord—have not shown responses to somatosensory stimuli (Figure 5–6; Kow and Pfaff, 1980). From these results, it appears that alterations in medullary reticular formation neuronal activity which prepare the way for lordosis must take place over a long period of time prior to the evocation of the behavioral response. Crucial reticulospinal activity is not of the spinobulbospinal reflex type, but must have a more tonic, preparatory nature.

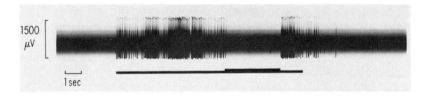

Figure 5–5. Responses of a neuron in the nucleus gigantocellularis of the medulla. Brushing of the hair on an area of skin of a female rat activated the unit. Concurrent pressure on the hindquarters inhibited it. (From Kow & Pfaff, 1980)

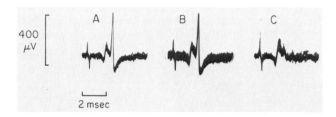

Figure 5–6. (A) Antidromic identification of a reticulospinal unit in the medulla of a female rat. Neuron is backfired from electrical stimulation of its axon in the ipsilateral lateral column of the spinal cord. (B) Antidromic response to stimulation at 50 per second. (C) After spinal cord hemisection, spike was absent even with 20× increase in stimulus. This cell did not respond to cutaneous stimulation. (From Kow & Pfaff, 1980)

2.   Midbrain

Somatosensory information that could be relevant for lordosis does reach midbrain neurons. Single unit activity was recorded with micropipettes from neurons in the dorsal midbrain of female rats lightly anesthetized with urethane (Malsbury, Kelley, and Pfaff, 1972). Single unit responses to cutaneous stimuli, including many on skin regions contacted by the male rat during mating, were recorded from neurons in and around the mesencephalic central gray (Table 5–2). Almost all responses were excitatory. No differences in midbrain cell responses to somatosensory input between untreated and hormone-primed female rats were detected (Malsbury et al., 1972).

However, the responses of midbrain cells to cutaneous stimulation probably do not tell the entire story, or even touch the main point of midbrain participation in the control of lordosis behavior. Subsequent recording experiments in urethane-anesthetized female rats included the antidromic identification of midbrain cells which project via descending axons to the reticular formation of the medulla (Sakuma and Pfaff, 1980b,c). Indeed, some neurons in and around the mesencephalic central gray responded convincingly to cutaneous stimuli. Typically, these neurons had wide receptive fields and, as in our previous work, virtually all responses were excitatory. Sensory responses were not changed in any obvious way by estrogen treatment (Sakuma and Pfaff, 1980d). Therefore, as our previous recording experiments showed, cutaneous information of the sort which triggers lordosis does reach midbrain neurons. However, those neurons whose responses would be most likely to direct lordosis behavior—the neurons whose axons descend to the medullary reticular formation—were virtually unresponsive. The best

Table 5-2. Responses of single midbrain units to somatosensory stimuli in female rats (Malsbury et al., 1972)

Type of unit	No.	Percent of all units	Percent of responsive units
"Touch units": skin location of receptive field			
Rear			
Areas touched by ♂	32	12	35
Other areas	6	2	7
Front	12	4	13
Whole body	15	6	16
"Painful pinch" units	27	10	29
Unresponsive units	178	66	—
Total	270	100	100

From Malsbury et al., 1972.

responses to somatosensory input came from neurons that were not antidromically identified (Figure 5–7). This finding raises the question of how powerful a role sensory input to the midbrain central gray could be in directing the behavior. Along the same lines, transection of ascending axons as they enter the mesencephalon may have no effect on lordosis behavior (Manogue et al., 1980a). Midbrain lesions placed to damage spinal–midbrain fibers as they head for the central gray do disrupt lordosis behavior, but central gray electrical stimulation can overcome the deficit (Sakuma and Pfaff, 1979). Thus, while sensory information for triggering lordosis can excite midbrain neurons, an important aspect of midbrain control over lordosis behavior must be an efferent signal that is not tightly locked to phasic sensory input and probably carries a hormone-dependent hypothalamic influence.

This is the highest level of the neuraxis at which the role of sensory information must be considered. Hypothalamic responses to reflex-triggering cutaneous input cannot be important for lordosis control (see Section E). Thalamic responses to sensory input are unlikely to be important, since spinothalamic axons can be severed without effect on female reproductive behavior (Manogue et al., 1980a). Subsequent chapters, therefore, treat the nature of hypothalamic (hormone-dependent) influences on the behavior control circuitry and the descending control over execution of the behavioral response.

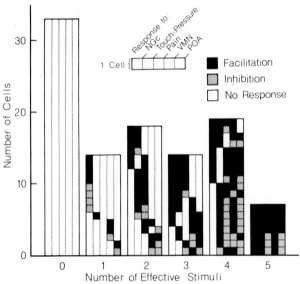

Figure 5–7. Patterns of response by neurons in or near midbrain central gray to somatosensory stimuli and other influences. These cells were *not* antidromically identified from the medulla. Neurons that *were* shown to have axons reaching the medulla did not respond to cutaneous stimuli. (From Sakuma & Pfaff, 1980d)

E. Hypothalamic Cells Not on the Sensory Side of the Reflex Loop

Does the hypothalamus participate in lordosis control through its responses to adequate lordosis-relevant somatosensory input? It appears not. We used micropipettes to record single unit activity of neurons in medial hypothalamic and medial preoptic regions that other evidence (Chapter 7) has implicated in the control of lordosis (Bueno and Pfaff, 1976). Only a small percentage of units responded to cutaneous stimuli that would trigger lordosis in unanesthetized hormone-primed female rats (Figure 5–8). Those unit responses that were detected were usually not very strong nor prompt. They would have to be immediate and strong responses to facilitate a reflex that begins about 160 milliseconds (Pfaff and Lewis, 1974) after the onset of stimulation.

Moreover, we expect that an important feature of hypothalamic participation in lordosis control is the estrogen dependence of its neuronal activity. From single unit recording (Bueno and Pfaff, 1976) we found that most of the estrogen-sensitive neurons in the hypothalamus fired very slowly, less than 1/second (Figure 5–9). The interspike intervals of such neurons, even during detectable responses to stimulation, are too long to facilitate lordosis (reflex latencies of less than 200 milliseconds) simply in response to immediate somatosensory input.

Other evidence also shows the rather slow nature of medial hypothalamic electrical activity. Facilitation of lordosis behavior in female rats by electrical stimulation in the ventromedial nucleus of the hypothalamus occurs with latencies typically between 25 and 50 minutes (Pfaff and Sakuma, 1979b). Unusually low frequencies of stimulation (less than 30/second) are required. Moreover, the effects of lesions of the same neurons on lordosis behavior take hours to appear (Pfaff and Sakuma, 1979a).

Thus, there is no strong evidence for the idea that, on each mount by the male rat, relevant somatosensory input ascends to the medial hypothalamus where neurons "make the decision" about lordosis according to the magnitude to their responses to this input. It appears that instead hypothalamic neurons participate in lordosis by a tonic hormone-dependent output, influencing the excitability of reflex loops completed at lower levels of the neuraxis (Chapters 7 and 8).

F. Summary and Implications

Some types of supraspinal facilitation is required for lordosis behavior. Critical pathways run in the anterolateral columns of the spinal cord. Insofar as ascending fibers participate in supraspinal lordosis control mechanisms, their impact on a subset of anterolateral system brainstem

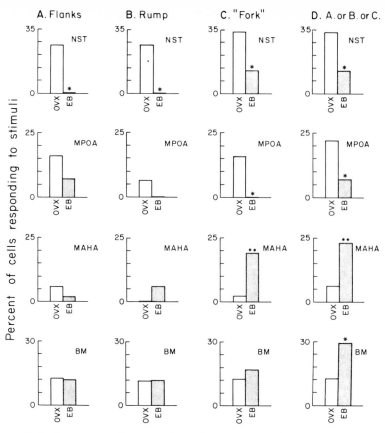

Figure 5–8. Percentage of neurons in each neuroanatomical structure responding to somatosensory stimuli. (A) Stimuli to the flanks. (B) Stimuli to the rump. (C) "Fork" stimuli, i.e., brief applications of pressure on the skin of the perineum, tailbase, and posterior rump. (D) Percentages of neurons that respond to at least one of the somatosensory stimuli shown in panels A, B, or C. Differences between responsiveness of neurons in estradiol-treated (*EB*) and untreated ovariectomized (*OVX*) female rat recording samples were statistically significant in some cases: *, $p < .05$; **, $p < .01$. *NST*, bed nucleus of stria terminalis; *MPOA*, medial preoptic area; *MAHA*, medial anterior hypothalamus; *BM*, basomedial hypothalamus. (From Bueno & Pfaff, 1976)

target sites must be considered. These sites are in the medullary reticular formation, the lateral vestibular nucleus, and, at midbrain levels, in and around the central gray. Some neurons in the medullary reticular formation and the midbrain central gray do respond to stimuli on lordosis-relevant skin areas. However, such responses may not be the essence of lordosis control. In the medullary reticular formation, antidromically identified reticulospinal cells do not respond, and cellular activity rates are not tightly, phasically locked to lordosis behavior. In the midbrain, also, neurons identified antidromically by their descending axons do not respond. Sensory control through the hypothalamus can be ruled out.

Therefore, descending facilitation of lordosis behavior by brainstem neurons is not simply the result of a spinal–brainstem–spinal reflex, triggering the behavior on a sensory-driven lordosis-by-lordosis basis. Thus, the sensory input must have its triggering action, lordosis by lordosis, at spinal levels (Figure 5–10). In turn, the facilitating role of

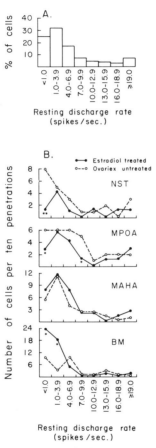

Figure 5–9. Distributions of resting discharge rates. (A) Distribution for all hypothalamic and preoptic neurons recorded in all rats. (B) Distributions for each anatomical structure plotted separately for estradiol-treated and untreated ovariectomized female rats. Numbers of neurons in each bin have been normalized according to the number of electrode penetrations through each anatomical structure. Differences between estradiol-treated and untreated female rat recording samples were statistically significant in some cases: *, $p < .05$; **, $p < .01$. Abbreviations as in Figure 5–8. (From Bueno & Pfaff, 1976)

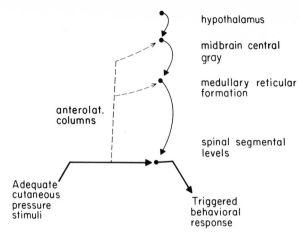

Figure 5–10. Logic of the neural pathways mediating sensory control over lordosis behavior. *Solid lines:* strong causal connections. *Broken lines:* neural connections for which anatomical evidence has been described, but which appear to be causally weak. Primary sensory triggering of lordosis behavior appears to occur at spinal levels. Ascending information arriving at medullary reticular neurons and midbrain central gray neurons is of more doubtful significance for lordosis-by-lordosis reflex control. Physiological mechanisms of medial hypothalamic cells are too slow to allow reflex triggering on a lordosis-by-lordosis basis.

descending fibers would have to be tonic in nature, in part reflecting estrogen influences that originate at the hypothalamus.

As a side point, note that the distribution of sensory information to various parts of the neural circuitry for lordosis seems to reflect, in the terms of an intelligence agency, the "need to know" principle. At higher levels of the circuitry, stimulus information does not need to be precise, in space or time. The modest role of information ascending to the brainstem appears to reflect great economy in the use of neurons (Chapter 12).

Part 2

Facilitating the Behavior:
Sex Hormones in the Brain

Chapter 6
Steroid Sex Hormone Binding by Cells in the Vertebrate Brain

A. Why Study Estrogen Binding?

Estrogen treatment followed by progesterone can induce behavioral sexual receptivity in ovariectomized female rodents (Beach, 1948; Young, 1961). In fact, estrogenic facilitation of female reproductive behavior has been found in a wide variety of vertebrate species (Crews and Silver, 1980; Kelley and Pfaff, 1978).

Over time, the optimal schedule of estrogen treatment for inducing reproductive behavior in ovariectomized female rats is as follows. Treatment with estradiol for a period of many days has a long-lasting preparatory effect in that it makes the animal more sensitive to subsequent estrogen treatment (Beach and Orndorff, 1974; Gerall and Dunlap, 1973; Parsons, Krieger, McEwan, and Pfaff, 1980a; Whalen and Nakayama, 1965). Following this long-term preparation by estrogen, a "priming" injection of estradiol is given to the ovariectomized female rat 40–50 hours before behavioral testing. Then progesterone is injected subcutaneously 2–8 hours before testing. Under these conditions of hormone treatment, females show high levels of reproductive behavior.

The minimum time needed between initial estrogen treatment and behavioral testing for the very beginning of lordosis facilitation is 16 hours (Green, Luttge, and Whalen, 1970; McEwen et al., 1975). When estrogen is applied over a long enough period (at least several days), it can facilitate behavioral receptivity in ovariectomized female rats without progesterone (Davidson, Rodgers, Smith, and Bloch, 1968; Pfaff, 1970b). Finally, relatively high doses of estrogen can partially substitute for progesterone in the final step of hormonal preparation (Kow and Pfaff, 1975a).

Estrogen can facilitate lordosis without circulating through the body, if it is administered directly in specific regions of the brain. Microimplants of estradiol, in small tubes have been used to help prove that behavioral effects of the hormone can be mediated by brain cells and to discover specific loci of hormone action. In the earliest experiments, 27-gauge tubes filled with estradiol and placed within the medial preoptic area activated feminine sexual behavior in ovariectomized female rats (Lisk, 1962). This finding has been replicated (Barfield and Chen, 1977; Chambers and Howe, 1968; Yanase and Gorski, 1976). However, an even more sensitive site for the local application of estradiol is the ventromedial nucleus of the hypothalamus (Dörner, Döcke, and Moustafa, 1968). Estrogen-filled 30-gauge tubes placed unilaterally in the ventromedial nucleus of the hypothalamus can activate lordosis behavior even when placements in the preoptic area or other sites give little or no behavioral facilitation (Barfield and Chen, 1977).

Chemical measurements of the radioactivity diffusing away from the hypothalamic estrogen implant site have shown that the hormone action really is local. With unilateral implants, radioactive hormone does not get to the other side of the hypothalamus and does not get, for instance, as far anterior as the preoptic area even when high levels of lordosis behavior have been stimulated (Davis, McEwen, and Pfaff, 1979). Similarly, autoradiography of hypothalamic tissue around sites of implantation of radioactive estradiol has shown a sharp gradient of hormone distribution away from the implant site (Davis, Krieger, and Pfaff, 1980). Therefore, it is clear that estrogen action on cells in the ventromedial region of the hypothalamus, and also in the medial preoptic area, can facilitate the hormone's effects on female reproductive behavior.

Pituitary action is not required for the induction of sex behavior by steroid hormones: estrogen and progesterone injections can cause lordosis in hypophysectomized ovariectomized female rats (Pfaff, 1970a). Likewise, pituitary hormones such as luteinizing hormone (LH) and follicle-stimulating hormone (FSH) have not been effective in facilitating rodent reproductive behavior (Moss and McCann, 1973; Pfaff, 1970a). Therefore, we have suspected that the facilitating effects of the hypothalamic decapeptide luteinizing hormone releasing factor (LRF) on reproductive behavior in female rats must be mediated by LRF effects in brain tissue (Moss and McCann, 1973; Pfaff, 1973).

In summary, estrogen followed by progesterone facilitates lordosis. It also has neuroendocrine effects such as triggering of the LH surge leading to ovulation. The behavioral effects of estrogen can operate through cells in the medial hypothalamus and medial preoptic area. This fits with the facts that spinally transected animals do not show estrogen-dependent behavior (Kow et al., 1977) and that single unit recording of sensory responses in the spinal cord has not shown marked estrogenic effects (Kow and Pfaff, 1979; Kow et al., 1980a). The failure of decerebrate female rats to show lordosis also suggests that hormone action above the level of the mesencephalon is required for lordosis behavior (Kow, Grill, and Pfaff, 1978). All of these facts are consistent with the notion that estrogen acts on hypothalamic cells, altering the activity of those cells in such a way as to facilitate female reproductive behavior. Thus, autoradiographic studies of radioactive estrogen accumulation by cells in the brain, especially the medial hypothalamus and medial preoptic area, have been especially important for delineating precise sites of hormone action.

B.   Estrogen Accumulation by Cells in Rat Central Nervous System

1.   Autoradiographic Studies

Using the technique of steroid hormone autoradiography for looking with high resolution through the light microscope at cellular accumulation of radioactive hormone, we have mapped the entire central nervous system of rats for the presence and location of estrogen-concentrating cells (Pfaff, 1968a; Pfaff and Keiner, 1973). Radioactive estrogen is concentrated specifically by cells in the medial preoptic area and certain cell groups in the medial hypothalamus (see below), in the limbic forebrain, and in a specific mesencephalic locus. In the limbic system, estrogen is accumulated by neurons in the medial and cortical amygdaloid nuclei, lateral septum, and (to a lesser extent) ventral hippocampus. A posterior extension of the estrogen-concentrating system is seen in the mesencephalon, where cells in the ventrolateral and dorsolateral portions of the midbrain central gray accumulate radioactive estradiol.

We are especially interested in estrogen concentration by cells that might be involved in the hormonal facilitation of lordosis. The locations of estrogen-concentrating cells are described in more detail below. We start in the medial preoptic area and proceed posteriorly through medial hypothalamic cell groups (Figure 6–1).

Cells in the medial preoptic area of female rats are heavily labeled with radioactive estradiol, especially near the midline at levels underneath the anterior commissure and in the preoptic area pars suprachiasmaticus. The lateral preoptic area is much less heavily labeled than the medial preoptic area, but it has a few labeled cells. The scattering of labeled cells there is similar to that at most levels of the medial forebrain bundle.

A large number of cells in the anterior hypothalamic area concentrate radioactive estradiol, especially, for instance, at levels just behind the anterior commissure but anterior to the paraventricular nucleus. Here, near the ventral border of the brain, many labeled cells are found near the third ventricle. Dorsally, this field of intensely labeled cells swings laterally away from the ventricle toward the descending fornix, stria medullaris, and stria terminalis. Further posterior, a high density of

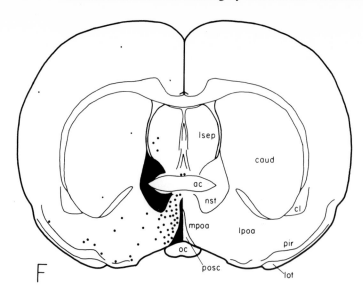

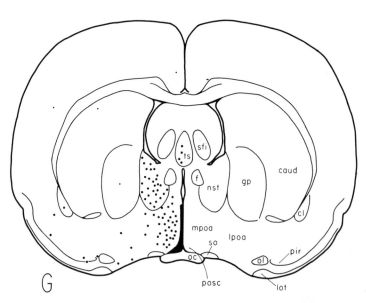

Figure 6–1. Preoptic and hypothalamic levels (F–O selected from an atlas) of estradiol-concentrating cells in the brain of the female rat. Locations of estradiol-concentrating cells found reliably at given sites are shown on the left side of the drawings (*large black dots*). Numbers of large black dots in a given region are roughly proportional to the number of estrogen-concentrating neurons, up to the highest density of labeled neurons; in these areas the density of labeled cells is so great that the black dots merge (*solid black areas*). In regions of very low uptake, scattered labeled cells can occasionally be seen, but not reliably in

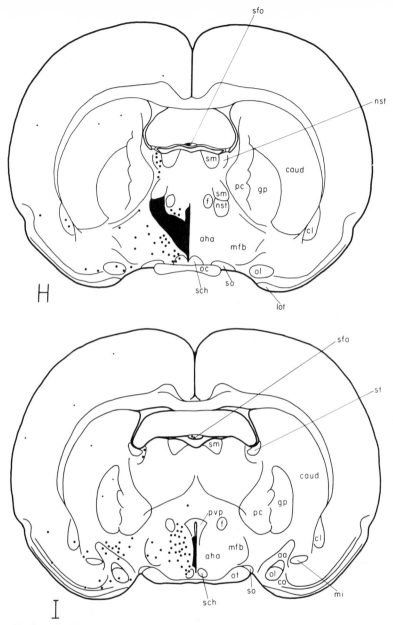

specific locations. (From Pfaff & Keiner, 1973) *Abbreviations: a,* nucleus accumbens; *aa,* anterior amygdaloid area; *ac,* anterior commissure; *aha,* anterior
hypothalamic area; *arc,* arcuate nucleus; *b,* basal amygdaloid complex; *bl,*
basolateral amygdaloid complex; *caud,* caudate nucleus; *cbllm,* cerebellum; *cc,*
corpus callosum; *ce,* central nucleus of the amygdala; *cg,* central gray; *cl,*
claustrum; *co,* cortical nucleus of the amygdala; *cp,* posterior commissure; *db,*
diagonal band of Broca; *dg,* dentate gyrus of the hippocampus; *dm,* dorsomedial
nucleus of the hypothalamus; *dpm,* dorsal premammillary nucleus of the hypo-

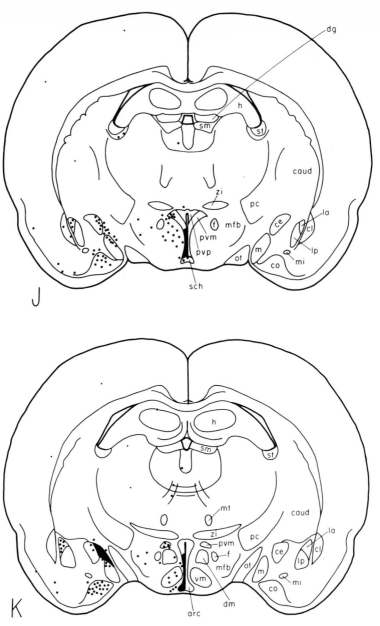

thalamus: *ent,* entorhinal cortex; *f,* fornix; *fr,* fasciculus retroflexus; *gp,* globus
pallidus; *h,* hippocampus; *ic,* inferior colliculus; *ICl,* island of Calleja; *icm,* island
of calleja magna; *ip,* interpeduncular nucleus; *la,* laternal nucleus of the amygdala
(pars anterior); *lc,* locus ceruleus; *lh,* lateral habenula; *lot,* lateral olfactory tract;
lp, lateral nucleus of the amygdala (pars posterior); *lpoa,* lateral preoptic area;
lsep (or ls), lateral septum; *m,* medial nucleus of the amygdala; *mamm,* mammillary bodies; *mch,* medial corticohypothalamic tract; *mcp,* middle cerebellar
peduncle; *mfb,* medial forebrain bundle; *mgb,* medial geniculate body; *mh,*

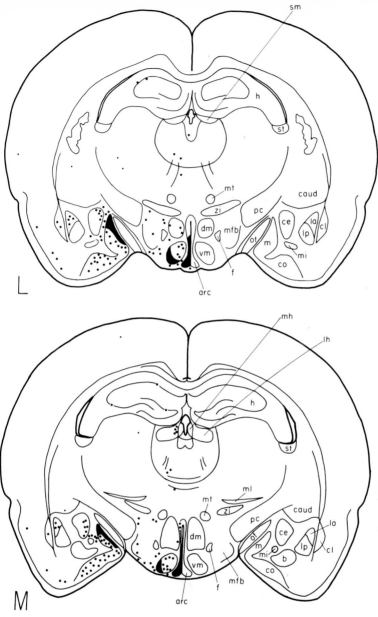

medial habenula; *mi*, massa intercalata; *ml*, medial lemniscus; *mlf*, medial longitudinal fasciculus; *mpoa*, medial preoptic area; *msep*, medial septum; *mt*, mammillothalamic tract; *mtg*, mammillotegmental tract; *nst*, bed nucleus of the stria terminalis; *ob*, olfactory bulb; *oc*, optic chiasm; *ol*, nucleus of the lateral olfactory tract; *on*, optic nerve; *ot*, optic tract; *pc*, cerebral peduncle; *perivent*, periventricular fibers; *pf*, nucleus parafascicularis; *pir*, prepiriform cortex; *posc*, preoptic area pars suprachiasmaticus; *pvm*, parventricular nucleus (magnocellular); *pvp*, paraventricular nucleus (parvicellular); *r*, red nucleus; *sc*, superior

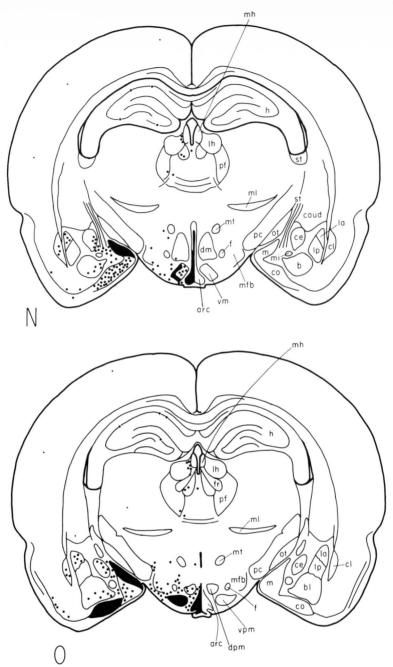

colliculus; *sch*, suprachiasmatic nucleus; *scp*, superior cerebellar peduncle; *sfi*, septofimbrial nucleus; *sfo*, subfornical organ; *sm*, stria medullaris; *so*, supraoptic nucleus; *sol*, superior olive; *st*, stria terminalis; *tb*, trapezoid body; *ts*, nucleus triangularis septi; *tub*, olfactory tubercle; *vc*, ventral cochlear nucleus; *vm*, ventromedial nucleus; *vpm*, ventral premammillary nucleus; *zi*, zona incerta; *III*, nucleus of the oculomotor nerve; *Vm*, mesencephalic nucleus of the trigeminal nerve; *Vs*, spinal nucleus of the trigeminal nerve; *tVs*, spinal tract of the trigeminal nerve.

labeling is found among the cells close to the third ventricle, between the paraventricular nucleus and the suprachiasmatic nucleus. The suprachiasmatic nucleus itself is virtually unlabeled. However, it is usually surrounded by estrogen-labeled cells on its dorsolateral and dorsomedial edges.

Estrogen-labeled cells in the paraventricular nucleus are found most reliably at the lateral caudal tip of the magnocellular part of this nucleus. Small cells just lateral to the paraventricular nucleus may also be labeled. The supraoptic nucleus is unlabeled.

High numbers of very heavily labeled cells are found after radioactive estradiol administration throughout the extent of the arcuate nucleus of the hypothalamus, from anterior hypothalamic levels through posterior levels that include the mammillary nuclei.

Estrogen-concentrating cells can be found throughout the extent of the ventromedial nucleus of the hypothalamus, especially in its ventrolateral subdivision. In many sections it is obvious that labeled cells are not restricted to well-defined borders of the nucleus. Estrogen-labeled cells can be found scattered medially toward the arcuate, dorsally toward the dorsomedial nucleus and fornix, and laterally along the bottom of the brain toward the lateral hypothalamic area (Figure 6–1).

Slightly more posterior, high numbers of estrogen-concentrating cells can be found throughout the ventral premammillary nucleus. Here also, in most sections, labeled cells are not restricted to the well defined borders of this nucleus, but are scattered laterally toward the posterior lateral hypothalamus. Lateral to this nucleus there regularly appears to be a field of estrogen-concentrating cells near the bottom of the brain.

The neuroanatomical distribution of estrogen-concentrating neurons described autoradiographically in the rat nervous system (Pfaff, 1968a; Pfaff and Keiner, 1973) does not represent an unspecific accumulation of chemicals in general or steroid hormones in particular. It is in striking contrast to the distribution of another functional steroid hormone, corticosterone (McEwen, Weiss, and Schwartz, 1969, 1970). Radioactive corticosterone is not accumulated specifically by cells in the preoptic area of medial hypothalamus, but instead is concentrated most highly by pyramidal cells in the hippocampus.

2.   Biochemical Studies

Cell fractionation studies of estrogen receptors in rat brain tissue have recently been summarized (McEwen, Davis, Parsons, and Pfaff, 1979). The neuroanatomical distribution of estrogen receptors as determined by isotope measurements of dissected brain tissue blocks in animals treated with tritiated estrogen agrees very well with the autoradiographic results described above (Eisenfeld and Axelrod, 1965, 1966; Kato and Villee, 1967a,b; McEwen and Pfaff, 1970; Zigmond and McEwen, 1970). In these biochemical studies as in autoradiography, high levels of estrogen accumulation are seen in the preoptic area, medial hypothalamus, and specific limbic structures. In addition, chemical studies show that specific receptors for estrogen exist in the cell nucleus (Zigmond and McEwen, 1970). Competition for receptors by nonradioactive estrogen proves that the receptors are of limited capacity. Estrogen receptors in brain tissue have a molecular size of about 8 S. These receptors have the greatest affinity for diethylstilbestrol, followed by the natural estrogen 17 β-est estradiol which in turn is much greater than the affinity for 17α-est estradiol (reviewed by McEwen, Davis, Parsons, and Pfaff, 1979). The specific accumulation of radioactive estrogen by limited capacity, energy using, stereospecific sites in the cytoplasm and nucleus of cells in the rat brain (which accumulation can be blocked by antiestrogens, as described below) is as expected for estrogen receptors in other estrogen-dependent tissues in the body (for instance, in the reproductive system, the uterus).

C.   Steroid Sex Hormone Binding by Cells in the Vertebrate Brain: From Fish to Philospher

In view of the complexity of the mammalian nervous system, it is of use to discover the most regular, evolutionarily stable, neuroanatomically lawful features of sex hormone binding by nerve cells. The anatomy of hormone binding in brain tissue may be more complicated than in other organs. With the types of electrical signaling networks found in brain, it is conceivable that individual neurons are uniquely arranged anatomically, and certainly small groups of neurons sometimes serve different functions than other small groups nearby. Indeed, it is for this reason that it has been essential to study hormone-binding neurons using autoradiography, which has histological resolution sufficient to identify individually labeled cell bodies. Thus, we have used steroid hormone autoradiography to study the accumulation of radioactive estradiol and testosterone by cells in the brains of a wide variety of vertebrate species, including all major vertebrate classes (Figure 6–2).

Our findings from bony fishes (Figure 6–3) and, as representatives of primates, rhesus monkeys (Figure 6–4) are summarized below. Estradiol and testosterone binding by cells in the brain is a phenomenon widespread among vertebrates. Certain cell groups in phylogenetically ancient parts of the forebrain, in the medial preoptic area and the medial hypothalamus, show up on all these cases as having steroid sex hormone–binding properties (Figure 6–5, Table 6–1).

For example, testosterone-concentrating cells in the brain of a teleost, the male green sunfish, have been investigated (Morrell, Kelley, and Pfaff, 1975a; report of unpublished findings by Morrell, Demski, and Pfaff). As expected, labeled cells were found in the medial preoptic area and in the tuberal region of the medial hypothalamus. More extensive

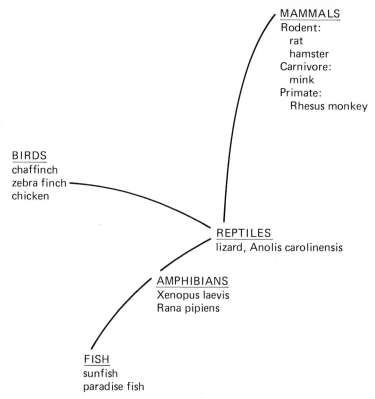

MAMMALS
Rodent:
  rat
  hamster
Carnivore:
  mink
Primate:
  Rhesus monkey

BIRDS
chaffinch
zebra finch
chicken

REPTILES
lizard, Anolis carolinensis

AMPHIBIANS
Xenopus laevis
Rana pipiens

FISH
sunfish
paradise fish

Figure 6–2. Vertebrate species studied in our laboratory for the neuroanatomical distribution of estrogen- or androgen-concentrating cells in the brain. [Recently, garter snakes (Halpern et al., 1980) have also been examined.] (From Pfaff & Conrad, 1978)

analyses of another type of fish, the male paradise fish (Davis, Morrell, and Pfaff, 1977), revealed the same type of neuroanatomical pattern of hormone binding, which was proving universal among vertebrates. Cells concentrating radioactive estradiol or testosterone in the brain of the paradise fish were found in the preoptic area, in tuberal cell groups in the medial hypothalamus (homologous to the arcuate nucleus), and in the ventral telencephalon (Figure 6–3; Davis et al., 1977).

As an example of our investigation at the other extreme of the vertebrate "phylogenetic tree" (Figure 6–2), we used autoradiography to locate and describe hormone-binding cells in the brain of adult female rhesus monkeys (Pfaff, Gerlach, McEwen, et al., 1976). Estrogen-binding cells were found in the medial preoptic area, medial anterior hypothalamus, ventromedial nucleus of the hypothalamus, and arcuate (infundibular) nucleus (Figure 6–4). In the limbic forebrain, cells in the bed nucleus of the stria terminalis and in the medial nucleus of the smygdala were well labeled. Some labeled cells were found in the ventral portions of the lateral septum. In contrast to this distribution of estrogen-labeled

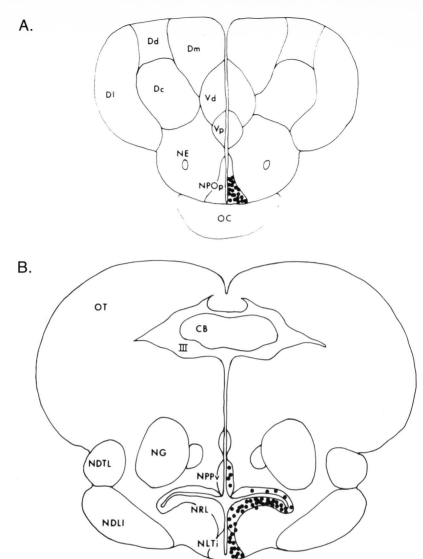

Figure 6-3 A and B. Locations of estrogen-concentrating cells in the brain of the paradise fish. (A) A section through the preoptic area (*NPOp*). (B) A section through hypothalamic nuclei in the tuberal (infundibular) region (*NRL, NLTi*). (From Davis et al., 1977)

cells, those that accumulated radioactive corticosterone were not found in the preoptic area of hypothalamus, but instead were in the hippocampus. Pyramidal neurons and dentate gyrus granule cells were labeled. Here, as in the rat, the different distributions of estrogen- and corticosterone-labeled cells prove specificity of hormone-binding processes in the brain (Pfaff et al., 1976). The neuroanatomical distributions shown by autoradiography were also seen in parallel biochemical experiments

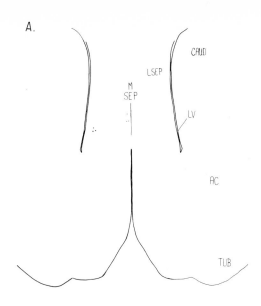

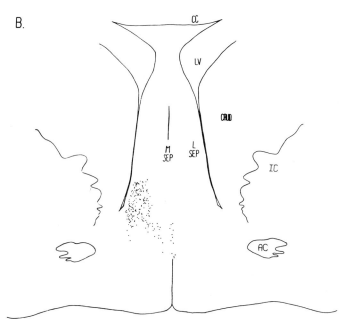

Figure 6–4. Charts from representative autoradiograms showing cells that concentrate ³H-estradiol in the basal forebrain and diencephalon of female rhesus monkeys. Precise locations of estradiol-labeled neurons are shown on the left-

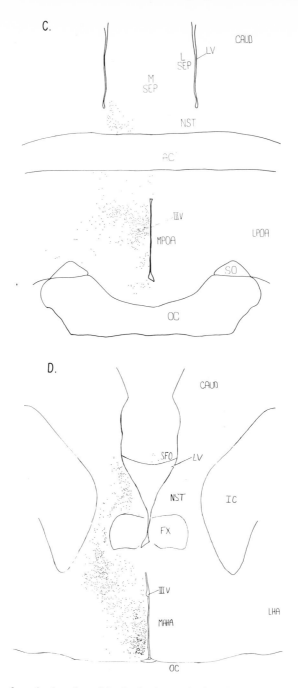

hand side of each drawing (*black dots*); each dot shows the position of one labeled cell body. *Broken line* (at the bottom of panel E): line where a block for the median eminence was separated. (From Pfaff et al., 1976) *Abbreviations: AC,* anterior commissure; *CAUD,* caudate nucleus; *CC,* corpus callosum; *CG,*

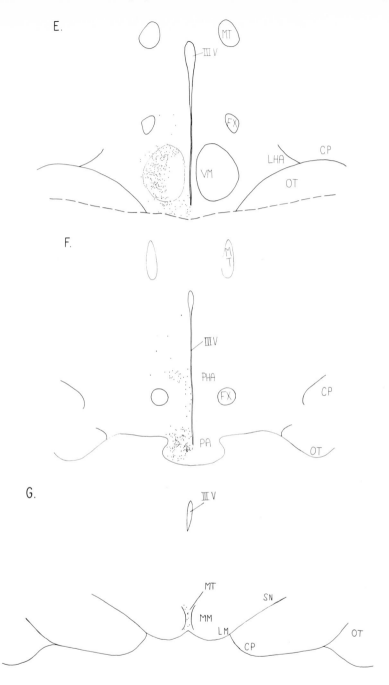

central gray; *CP*, cerebral peduncle; *FX*, fornix; *HI*, habenulointerpeduncular tract; *IC*, internal capsule; *LHA*, lateral hypothalamic area; *LM*, lateral mammillary nucleus; *LPOA*, lateral preoptic area; *LSEP*, lateral septum; *LV*, lateral ventricle; *MAHA*, medial anterior hypothalamus; *MM*, medial mammillary

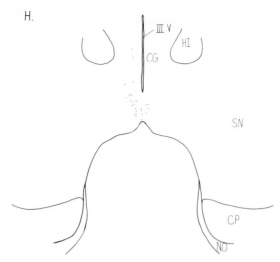

nucleus; *MPOA*, medial preoptic area; *MSEP*, medial septum; *MT*, mammillothalamic tract; *NO*, oculomotor nerve; *NST*, bed nucleus of stria terminalis; *OC*,
optic chiasm; *OT*, optic tract; *PA*, posterior arcuate (infundibular) nucleus; *PHA*,
posterior hypothalamic area; *SFO*, subfornical organ; *SN*, substantia nigra; *SO*,
supraoptic nucleus; *TUB*, olfactory tubercle; *VM*, ventromedial nucleus of
hypothalamus; *IIIV*, third ventricle.

with rhesus monkeys (Gerlach, McEwen, Pfaff, et al., 1976); they proved
estrogen binding by cell nuclei in the hypothalamus and corticosterone
binding by cell nuclei in the hippocampus.

Certain features of the neuroanatomy of estrogen and androgen binding
by cells in the brain appear to be general across all vertebrates (Pfaff,
1976). This phylogenetic survey (Figure 6–2) has included paradise fish
(Davis et al., 1977), sunfish (Morrell et al., 1975a), the amphibians
Xenopus laevis (Kelley, Morrell, and Pfaff, 1975; Kelley and Pfaff, 1976;
Morrell et al., 1975a) and *Rana pipiens* (Kelley, Lieberburg, McEwen,
and Pfaff, 1978), and, among reptiles, the lizard *Anolis carolinensis*
(Morrell et al., 1977a, 1979) and the garter snake (Halpern, Morrell, and
Pfaff, 1980). Among birds, we have studied the chaffinch (Zigmond,
Detrick, and Pfaff, 1980; Zigmond, Nottebohm, and Pfaff, 1973), the
zebra finch (Arnold, Nottebaum, and Pfaff, 1976), and the chicken
(Barfield, Ronay, and Pfaff, 1978). The mammals we have studied
include, among rodents, the rat (Pfaff, 1968a,b; Pfaff and Keiner, 1973)
and hamster (Krieger, Morrell, and Pfaff, 1976); among carnivores, the
mink (Morrell, Ballin, and Pfaff, 1977a,b); and among primates, the
rhesus monkey (Gerlach et al., 1976; Pfaff et al., 1976).

In all of these cases (Table 6–1) we were able to find estrogen- or
androgen-binding nerve cells in specific locations. Hormone-concentrating cells were always found in the medial preoptic area, in medial
hypothalamic cell groups, and in specific limbic forebrain structures

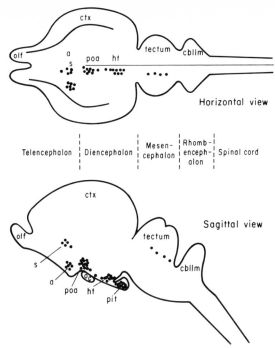

Figure 6–5. Abstract representation of a "generalized vertebrate brain," showing locations of estradiol- and testosterone-concentrating neurons common to all vertebrates studied thus far. *Black dots:* groups of steroid-concentrating cells. Features of the distribution of ^{3}H-estradiol and ^{3}H-testosterone that are common across vertebrates include labeled cells in the limbic telencephalon (e.g., septum, amygdala, or archistriatum), preoptic area, tuberal hypothalamic nuclei, and specific subtectal loci in the mesencephalon. Nauta and Karten (1970) was used as a reference for the generalized view of the vertebrate brain. *a,* amygdala or archistriatum; *cbllm,* cerebellum; *ctx,* cortex (nonmammalian, general cortex; mammalian, neocortex); *ht,* nuclei in tuberal region of hypothalamus; *oc,* optic chiasm; *olf,* olfactory bulb; *pit,* pituitary; *poa,* preoptic area; *s,* septum; *tectum* (nonmammalian, optic tectum and inferior colliculus; mammalian, superior colliculus and inferior colliculus). (From Morrell & Pfaff, 1977)

Table 6-1. Results of Autoradiographic Studies of Steroid Sex Hormone–Binding Cells in the Brains of Vertebrates

1. All species have hormone-concentrating nerve cells in specific locations.
2. Hormone-concentrating cells are in the medial preoptic area, medial (tuberal) hypothalamus, and limbic forebrain structures.
3. Nerve cell groups that bind hormones participate in the control of hormone-modulated functions.

Note. These features are common to all species studied.
From Pfaff & Conrad, 1978.

(Figure 6–5). Finally, when the autoradiographic distributions of hormone-concentrating cells were compared with the experimental physiology of each species in question, it was obvious that nerve cell groups
that bind estrogen or androgen participate in the control of steroid
hormone–modulated functions.

The correlations of hormone binding with the location of nerve cells
controlling hormone-dependent functions were obvious in the cases of
medial preoptic and medial hypothalamic nerve cells, which have been
shown to control mating behavior, and tuberal hypothalamic cell groups,
which have been shown to control gonadotropin release. Even in subtler
cases, involving certain intersting additions to the general neuroanatomical vertebrate pattern of hormone binding, the correlations between
hormone-binding nerve cells and hormone-dependent neural controls
held up perfectly (Kelley and Pfaff, 1978). For example, in the zebra
finch (Arnold et al., 1976), cells of nucleus MAN and the neostriatum,
the caudal nucleus of the hyperstriatum ventrale, and the tracheosyringealis portion of the hypoglossal nucleus of the medulla concentrate
androgen. Lesion studies and subsequent neuroanatomical work have
shown the same nerve cell groups are involved in the control of song
(Nottebohm, Stokes, and Leonard, 1976), which in these birds depends
on androgenic hormones. The tracheosyringealis portion of the hypoglossal nucleus is especially interesting, because it contains cells whose
axons innervate the musculature responsible for producing bird song. In
the frog *Xenopus laevis* (Kelley et al., 1975; Morrell et al., 1975a) the
uptake of androgen but not estrogen was demonstrated by cells in a
motor cranial nerve nucleus (IX–X). These cells have been postulated to
control androgen-dependent frog vocalizations (Schmidt, 1974). Many
points of the neural circuitry for the control of frog reproductive behavior
(Schmidt, 1974) overlap with the distribution of androgen-concentrating
cells as shown by autoradiography. Spatial correlations between steroid-
concentrating nerve cells and the neural circuitry for hormone-dependent
behavioral responses (both those general across vertebrates and those
particular as described above) strengthen our suspicion that hormone
binding by nerve cells represents the first step in the control of behavior
by steroid sex hormones.

D.   Combinations of Steroid Hormone Autoradiography with Other Histochemical Identification Techniques

With the locations of estrogen-concentrating cells in the brain of the
female rat so well described, what else can we discover about the identity
of these cells? Using the retrograde transport technique of neuroanatom-

ical pathway tracing, with horseradish peroxidase, we have applied HRP
to the central gray of the midbrain and processed hypothalamic tissue
sections for combined visualization of HRP and estradiol autoradiography
(Morrell and Pfaff, 1980). We have never seen an overlap of HRP
(transported retrograde to the cell body) and radioactive estrogen on the
same hypothalamic cell (Figure 6–6). This lack of overlap between
estrogen-concentrating cells and cells projecting to the midbrain central
gray is striking, since we know (see below) that axons of hypothalamic
cells mediating estrogen-dependent reproductive behavior end in and
near the central gray. Using immunohistochemical techniques for the
visualization of neurophysins applied to tissue also processed for estrogen
autoradiography, we have been able to see neurophysins and radioactive
estrogens in the same cell bodies in the paraventricular nucleus (Figure
6–7; Morrell, Rhodes, and Pfaff, 1980). This is interesting because it had
been previously demonstrated that estrogen can stimulate the production
and release of one class of neurophysins. Current work in the laboratory
will compare the cell-by-cell distribution of radioactive estrogen and
LRF.

   To date, we have no evidence that estrogen-containing cells project
other than locally. If these trends are generally true, then we would have
to conclude that estrogen affects the chemical and electrical output of
the medial hypothalamus through a system of estrogen-addressed local
interneurons.

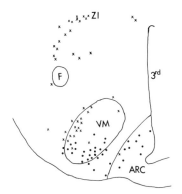

Figure 6–6. Results of the combined steroid autoradiographic–HRP retrograde
tracing method in rat hypothalamic cells. *Black dots:* individual ³H-estradiol-
labeled cells with black grains visible over the nucleus of the cell. *Crosses:*
individual retrogradely labeled, HRP-containing cells, with blue-black TMB
reaction product visible over the soma and cellular processes, but not over the
nucleus. No single cell has both HRP and ³H-estradiol label, although cells
labeled with either exist next to one another. All the labeled cells found in a
single 14-μm section (one side) are represented here. This is a transverse section
through the medial–basal hypothalamus. Dorsal is toward the top, lateral toward
the left. *ARC,* arcuate nucleus; *VM,* ventromedial nucleus; *F,* fornix; *3ʳᵈ,* third
ventricle; *ZI,* zona incerta. (From Morrell & Pfaff, 1980)

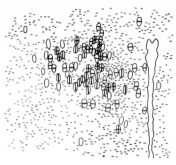

Figure 6–7. Camera lucida drawing of a 6-μm section through a portion of the paraventricular nucleus of the rat showing the results of the combination of the steroid autoradiographic technique with the immunocytochemical technique (Rhodes, Morrell & Pfaff, in preparation). The steroid autoradiogram (^{3}H-estradiol) was exposed for 4 months; the immunocytochemistry was done for neurophysin (Bovine I primary antibody). A cresyl violet counterstain was used. Dorsal is at the top, the third ventricle is at the right; this is a transverse section.◯, Magnocellular cells;   , all other cells; ◯, cells with neurophysin in their cytoplasm; ◯, cells with ^{3}H-estradiol concentrated in the nucleus; ◯, cells with *both* neurophysin staining and ^{3}H-estradiol concentration. (From Morrell, Crews, Ballin, Morgentaler, & Pfaff, 1979)

E. Effects of Estrogen in the Hypothalamus

1. Morphological Effects

Since cells in and around the ventromedial nucleus of the hypothalamus have a high affinity for estradiol and (from the implant evidence cited above) probably mediate estrogen effects on female reproductive behavior, we studied their cellular architecture using electron microscopy (Cohen and Pfaff, 1979, 1980). Estradiol was subcutaneously injected daily in one group of ovariectomized female rats, while the control group was injected only with the oil vehicle. After 20 days of exposure to estrogen, the rats in the experimental group showed strong lordosis reflexes, while the control animals showed no lordosis at all. Hypothalamic and other brain tissue was prepared for electron microscopy with conventional procedures (Peters, Palay, and Webster, 1970).

Sections through the ventrolateral portion of the ventromedial nucleus of the hypothalamus showed that it consists mainly of neurons with a few interspersed glial cells. The neurons contain large oval nuclei, the nuclear membrane of which is often invaginated; the nucleoplasm is finely granular with a densely granular nucleolus. The assemblage of organelles present includes rough endoplasmic reticulum, a Golgi complex with coated vesicles attached or in the vicinity, small (about 125-nm) dense-core vesicles, lysosomelike bodies, dense granular non-membrane bound structures referred to as inclusion bodies, multivesicular bodies, and occasionally myelin figures (Figures 6–8 and 6–9).

Two differences seen in the ventrolateral portion of the ventromedial nucleus of the hypothalamus between estrogen treated and untreated overiectomized females were that the estrogen treated animals had a greater stacking of rough endoplasmic reticulum and a greater number of dense-core vesicles (Table 6–2). King, Williams, and Gerall (1973) also found changes in the organization of the rough endoplasmic reticulum and dense-core vesicles in neurons of the arcuate nucleus of the hypothalamus of female rats during the estrous cycle. The changes we have seen indicate greater biosynthetic and/or secretory activity in these ventromedial hypothalamic cells in the estrogen-treated than in the control animals.

2. Electrophysiological Effects

The electrical activity of hypothalamic units varies during the estrous cycle of the female rat (Cross and Dyer, 1971; Dyer, 1973; Dyer, Pritchett, and Cross, 1972; Kawakami, Terasawa, and Obuki, 1970; Moss and Law, 1971; Terasawa and Sawyer, 1969; see Pfaff, 1973b, for a

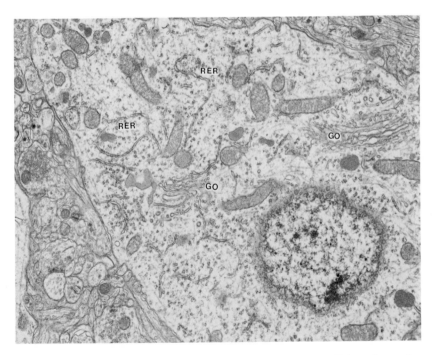

Figure 6–8. Electron micrograph of a cell in the ventromedial nucleus of an ovariectomized rat treated with sesame oil. Cisternae of the rough endoplasmic reticulum (*RER*) occur singly and are dispersed. No dense-cored vesicles are seen in the region of the Golgi complex (*GO*). ×25,000. (Data from Cohen & Pfaff, 1979, 1980)

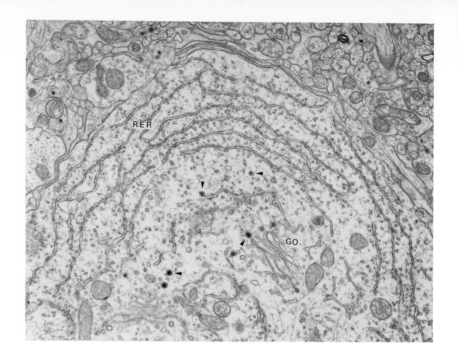

Figure 6–9. Electron micrograph of a cell in the ventromedial nucleus of an ovariectomized rat treated with estrogen. Cisternae of the rough endoplasmic reticulum (*RER*) are stacked in regular arrays. Numerous dense-core vesicles (*arrowheads*) are seen in the region of the Golgi complex (*GO*). ×25,000. (Data from Coehn & Pfaff, 1979, 1980)

Table 6-2. Electron microscopic demonstration of morphological effects of estrogen on nerve cells in the ventrolateral subdivision of the ventromedial nucleus of the female rat hypothalamus

Nerve cells with stacked ER[a] (%)				Dense-core vesicles (per 10 nerve cells sampled)			
Estrogen-treated		Control[c]		Estrogen-treated		Control[c]	
Rat No.		Rat No.		Rat No.		Rat No.	
1	53	1'	11	1	21.4	1'	15.0
2	28	2'	13	2	10.0	2'	6.0
3	46	3'	6	3	34.4	3'	1.1
4	44	4'	28	4	15.4	4'	3.3
5	43	5'	18	5	17.2	5'	6.3
6	29	6'	21	6	5.8	6'	2.4
MEAN	40.5[b]		16.2[b]		17.4[b]		5.7[b]

[a]ER: endoplasmic reticulum.

[b]Estrogen-treated versus control, $p < .02$.

[c]Ovariectomized, untreated rats.

Data from Cohen & Pfaff, 1979, 1980.

review). Variations during the estrous cycle might reflect the effects of estrogen. However, since blood levels of several hormones (both steroid hormones and pituitary hormones) change simultaneously during the estrous cycle, individual manipulations of estrogen alone have been required for a clear analysis of the effects of that hormone.

In one experiment electrical activity of single neurons was recorded with micropipettes in the medial hypothalamus and preoptic area of urethane-anesthetized ovariectomized female rats, some treated with estrogen and others untreated (Bueno and Pfaff, 1976). A comparison of the two groups showed that in the medial preoptic region and bed nucleus of the stria terminalis, estrogen-treated rats had fewer cells with recordable spontaneous activity, due primarily to a loss of cells with very slow firing rates (Figure 5–9); in the medial hypothalamic region in and around the ventromedial nucleus, estrogen-treated rats had more cells (than untreated rats) with recordable spontaneous activity, due primarily to a reappearance of cells with very slow firing rates (Figure 5–9). Estrogen treatment depressed responsiveness to somatosensory stimulation in the medial preoptic neurons and neurons in the bed nucleus of the stria terminalis, while it tended to elevate that in the neurons in the medial anterior hypothalamus and basal medial hypothalamus (in and around the ventromedial nucleus) (Figure 5–8).

At first the difference in the direction of the estrogen effect between preoptic and ventromedial hypothalamic neurons was surprising. However, upon reexamining the literature, we found that previous studies also had shown such differences, although they had not been pointed out. Terasawa, Ibuki, and Manaka (1971) found increases in the firing rate of arcuate neurons following estrogen treatment. Cross and Dyer (1972) found increases in the medial anterior hypothalamus. In spayed female cats, responsiveness in the ventromedial nucleus and the medial anterior hypothalamus was greater following estrogen treatment, and there was a shift in the direction of response toward excitation (Alcaraz, Guzman-Flores, Salas, and Beyer, 1969). In contrast, among neurons in the medial preoptic area, Whitehead and Ruf (1974) and Yagi (1970, 1973; Yagi and Sawaki, 1973) found units that decreased their resting discharge rates to very low levels for a long time after estrogen administration. Likewise, Kelly, Moss, and Dudley (1976) found that microelectrophoresed estradiol had predominantly inhibitory effects on medial preoptic neurons in female rats. Lincoln (1967) found that long-term estrogen treatment of ovariectomized rats was followed by lower spontaneous activity of preoptic units, units at the very anterior border of the medial anterior hypothalamus, and units in the lateral septum. Responses of preoptic neurons to probing of the vaginal cervix were shifted significantly in the direction of inhibition following estrogen treatment (Lincoln and Cross, 1967).

Thus, estradiol has significant electrophysiological effects on nerve cells in the same brain regions where it is bound. Moreover, after systemic estrogen treatment, there are stable differences in the nature of the hormone effect between preoptic and basomedial hypothalamic neurons. Interestingly, there are parallel differences in the neurochemical effects of estrogen between preoptic and basomedial hypothalamic regions (Luine and McEwen, 1980). Most important, the difference between the electrophysiological effect of estrogen in the preoptic neurons and that in the basomedial hypothalamic neurons matches perfectly the difference between the effects of these two neural regions on lordosis behavior in female rats (Chapter 7).

Electrophysiological effects of estrogen presumably are based on hormone-caused neurochemical alterations. Therefore, it is interesting that neurochemical effects of long-term estrogen administration have been reported, and that the nature of these effects is different in the preoptic region than in the basomedial hypothalamus (Luine and McEwen, 1980). Following estrogen binding, a behaviorally important estrogen effect depends on RNA synthesis. Infusion of actinomycin D into the preoptic area of estrogen-treated female rats can block estrogen-stimulated lordosis behavior (Hough, Cook, and Quadango, 1974; Quadagno, Shryne, and Gorski, 1971; Whalan, Gorzalka, DeBold, et al., 1974). Thus, the electrophysiological effects of estrogen on preoptic and hypothalamic neurons are accompanied by neurochemical effects, including biosynthetic steps important for the eventual behavioral effect of the hormone.

F.   Implications of the Estrogen-Binding Processes

1.   Correlations of Estrogen-Binding with Effects on Reproductive Behavior

The net result of the action of estrogen in the brain is a sequence of orderly changes in pituitary function and behavior. The ultimate purpose of many of the experiments noted above is to show a causal sequence of events, leading from estrogen entry into the brain and its accumulation by specific receptors to the final alterations in individual nerve cell activity which cause reproductive behaviors to occur. However, the information necessary for the construction of such a sequence is still lacking. At present, our investigation of how estrogen receptors are related to behavioral mechanisms is limited to the study of correlations between receptor function and behavioral function. Three types of correlations have been found: (a) those based on neuroanatomical studies of estrogen receptors and behavioral mechanisms (correlations in space); (b) those based on the temporal properties of estrogen action (temporal correlations); and (c) those based on the fact that antiestrogens can block both estrogen accumulation and estrogen effects on mating behavior (correlations of antiestrogen effects).

a. Spatial correlations. In the female rat brain, estradiol is concentrated by cells in the same neuroanatomical regions where estrogens can facilitate lordosis behavior. Studies have shown that microimplants of estrogen in and around the ventromedial nucleus of the hypothalamus, as well as in the medial preoptic area, facilitate female reproductive behavior (see Section A). Radioactive estradiol is bound by cells in exactly the same regions (Pfaff and Keiner, 1973; see Section B).

b. Temporal correlations. In general, very fast hormonal effects (within a few seconds or less) may not depend upon the types of cellular estrogen receptors described above. Slower actions of estrogen (taking a few hours or more) generally are thought to allow time for the hormone to enter the nucleus and alter genomic expression, with subsequent changes in biosynthetic events. The effects of estrogen on female rodent reproductive behavior are slow. Beginning with the longest-term estrogen action, Beach and Orndorff (1974), Gerall and Dunlap (1973) and Whalen and Nakayama (1965) showed that animals that had received estrogen over a period of many days or weeks were more sensitive to subsequent estrogen treatment. Subsequent experiments in our laboratory, which employed implants of estradiol to overcome certain technical reservations about the earlier studies, confirmed this conclusion (Parsons, Krieger, McEwen, and Pfaff, 1980). In studying the period of estrogen action that prepares the female rat for final progesterone injection and behavioral testing, Green et al. (1970) could find no estrogenic facilitation of female reproductive behavior less than 16 hours after an intravenous estradiol injection. After that, a gradual increase in receptivity was seen, until maximal behavioral receptivity appeared at hour 24. Similarly, we found that even in ovariectomized female rats that had been given a long-term estrogen preparatory treatment that final estrogen effect took more than 20 hours to register convincingly (McEwen et al., 1975). Since these females had been given a behaviorally effective intravenous injection of ^{3}H-estradiol, we were able to see that, while considerable nuclear occupation by radioactive estradiol was present 4 hours after hormone administration, little or no labeled estrogen was found in the brain at the time (after 20 hours) that behavioral responses began to occur. Thus, after long-term preparatory and priming action by estrogen, the estradiol does not actually have to be present in the brain at the time of behavioral testing for its effect on reproductive behavior to occur. These results are consistent with the idea that due to a time-consuming process of estrogen reception and subsequent estrogen-stimulated biosynthetic activity, a train of chemical events is triggered in behaviorally relevant hypothalamic neurons which does not need the further presence of estrogen for its completion. In fact, many biochemical effects of estrogen in the hypothalamus are only observed hours after estradiol administration (Table 7 in McEwen, Davis, Parsons, and Pfaff, 1979). Altogether, the effects of estradiol on female rat reproductive behavior, and some of the hypothalamic biochemical effects, are slow enough to allow time for binding of the hormone in the cytoplasm and then the nucleus, and for subsequent alterations in cellular biosynthetic activity.

c. Antiestrogens block estrogen-binding and estrogen-stimulated reproductive behavior. Studies showing the results of decreased estrogen-binding have recently been reviewed by McEwen, Davis, Parsons, and Pfaff (1979). A group of compounds classified as antiestrogens block the nuclear binding of estradiol in the uterus (Capony and Rochefort, 1975; Ruh and Ruh, 1974). Antiestrogens (for example, CI-628) can also block accumulation of radioactive estradiol in cell nuclei in the brain (Chazal, Faudon, Gogan, and Rotsztejn, 1975; Luine and McEwen, 1977; Luttge, Gray, and Hughes, 1976; Roy and Wade, 1977).

Antiestrogens prevent the long-term uterine responses to estradiol which provide estrogen-stimulated uterine growth (Katzenellenbogen and Ferguson, 1975), presumably by interfering with the nuclear action of an estrogen–receptor complex (Buller and O'Malley, 1976). Comparisons among the uterine growth responses following treatment with estradiol, estriol, and long-acting estriol derivatives have shown marked differences in the effectiveness of these various compounds. These differences are related to the duration of binding of these various steroids (Anderson, Peck, and Clark, 1975; Lan and Katzenellenbogen, 1976). Can parallel effects of antiestrogens on binding and function be shown in studies with estrogen-stimulated mating behavior?

Indeed, systemic injections of antiestrogens diminished estrogen-stimulated lordosis behavior. Decreased lordosis follows the blocking action of CI-628 (Arai and Gorski, 1968; Powers, 1975; Roy and Wade, 1977) and clomiphene (Ross, Paup, Brant-Zawadski, et al., 1973). Similar results also follow treatment with the antiestrogen MER-25 (Meyerson and Lindstrom, 1968).

Thus, both in peripheral and nervous tissue, decreased estrogen binding is correlated with decreased estrogen action. In brain tissue, this includes decreased estrogen stimulation of female mating behavior. It is reasonable to conclude that estrogen binding in brain tissue is necessary for normal estrogenic stimulation of lordosis behavior.

d. Reasoning. On spatial grounds, with neuroanatomical studies, on temporal grounds, with behavioral studies, and on pharmacological grounds, with antiestrogen studies, estrogen-binding phenomena in the brain are correlated with estrogen-stimulated lordosis behavior. It is reasonable to assume that binding of estrogen by hypothalamic cells, first in the cytoplasm and then in the cell nucleus, comprises an important set of steps eventually leading to behavioral effects.

2. Temporal Properties of Hypothalamic Participation

All aspects of the estrogenic control of lordosis, routed through the hypothalamus, appear to be slow acting. The hormone effect itself is slow (see above). Estrogen preparation can remain effective over weeks (Parsons, Krieger, McEwen, and Pfaff, 1980). The final priming action of estrogen takes no less than 16 hours (Green et al., 1970), with maximum responses not reached until after 24 hours (McEwen et al., 1975). Electrical activity of cells in the hypothalamus is also slow. Among neurons that have appeared to be estrogen sensitive (Bueno and Pfaff, 1976), resting discharge was absent or less than 1/p second, and there were no prompt, vigorous responses to somatosensory input. Reflecting these electrophysiological properties, the effects of hypothalamic cells on lordosis are slow. Minimum latencies of the electrically stimulated facilitation of lordosis from the ventromedial nucleus of the hypothalamus are 25–50 minutes, and unusually low frequencies of electrical stimulation are required for this effect (Pfaff and Sakuma, 1979b). Even the effects of ventromedial hypothalamic lesions on lordosis behavior take hours to develop (Pfaff and Sakuma, 1979a). Each of these temporal properties provide evidence against the notion that hypothalamic cells participate in a fast acting reflex loop, for instance, by virtue of their fast responses to somatosensory input. All facts appear consistent with the notion of a tonic estrogen-dependent output from the hypothalamus that affects the excitability of lordosis-relevant reflex loops completed at lower levels of the neuraxis.

3. Aspects of Estrogen-Sensitive Neurons: Preliminary Ideas

We know that estrogen-sensitive hypothalamic mechanisms register their effect on lordosis behavior by projections to the midbrain, ending in and around the central gray (see below). Nevertheless, the projection of hypothalamic cells that also accumulate estrogen in and around the central gray has not yet been demonstrated by the combined use of estrogen autoradiography and HRP histochemical techniques (Section D). If this evidence is generally correct, then estrogen-sensitive cells in the hypothalamus do not have their effects on the central gray by projecting there directly, but rather act as local interneurons, altering the activity of nearby neurons that do project to the midbrain central gray.

G.   Summary

Estrogen- and androgen-concentrating neurons have been found in specific locations in the brains of all vertebrate species. In all cases, specific cell groups in the medial hypothalamus (around the pituitary stalk), medial preoptic area, and limbic forebrain have steroid sex hormone-binding properties. For each species it is possible to document strong anatomical correlations between the locations of estrogen- or androgen-binding cells and the control of steroid-dependent pituitary or behavioral functions.

In the brain of the female rat, strong concentrations of estrogen-binding cells in the ventromedial nucleus of the hypothalamus, as well as in the anterior hypothalamus and medial preoptic area, are especially relevant to the control of lordosis behavior. In the ventrolateral subdivision of the ventromedial nucleus of the hypothalamus, estrogen causes changes in cellular architecture which indicate increased biosynthetic and/or secretory activity. The electrophysiological effects of estrogen on cells in this region are most apparent in nuerons that fire very slowly. The idea that estrogen binding by cells there leads to these effects and thence to lordosis behavior is supported by a set of correlations: spatial, neuroanatomical correlations between sites of estrogen binding and sites of estrogen action on lordosis behavior; temporal correlations related to the slow actions of estrogenic hormones in hypothalamic cells on lordosis behavior; and correlations based on the fact that antiestrogens can block estrogen binding in the brain and affect estrogen-dependent reproductive behavior.

Estrogen binding by cells in and around the ventromedial nucleus of the hypothalamus (Figure 6–10), over a period of at least 16 hours and usually including many days, leads to increased biosynthetic activity in

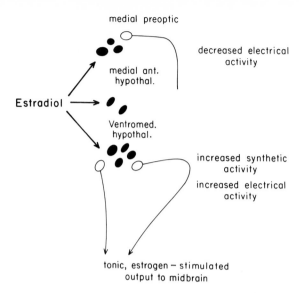

Figure 6–10. Summary of estrogen impact on hypothalamus, as related to cellular mechanisms of lordosis behavior.

these cells. One result of this is increased electrical activity in slowly firing cells in this region. The eventual result is an increased tonic estrogen-dependent output to the midbrain which facilitates lordosis behavior.

Chapter 7

Hypothalamic Mechanisms

A. Participation by Hypothalamic Cells in the Control of Lordosis

The most important input to hypothalamic cells for the control of lordosis appears to be hormonal (Chapter 6). Since lordosis is strongly controlled by estrogen in female rats, estrogenic influences on hypothalamic cells are considered primary. In fact, in a wide variety of vertebrate species, estrogens restore sexual receptivity to castrated females (Kelley and Pfaff, 1978). The accumulation of radioactive estradiol by hypothalamic nerve cells in female rats, as well as in a wide variety of vertebrate species (see Chapter 6), has shown possible sites of estrogenic action in controlling female reproductive behavior. Electron microscopic and electrophysiological results have shown estrogen effects on cells in hypothalamic regions where estrogen is bound. Finally, direct implantation of estrogen into the ventromedial nucleus of the hypothalamus or the medial preoptic area allows the performance of female reproductive behavior by ovariectomized female rats.

Thus, the hormonal influences of estrogen on these cells are likely to be strong. In turn, from the arguments in previous chapters, it appears that immediate hypothalamic neuronal responses in cutaneous input do not govern reflex performance of lordosis. We have concluded that the hypothalamus should not be conceived of as lying on the "ascending side" of the obligatory supraspinal lordosis control loop; rather, hormonal input to hypothalamic tissue alters hypothalamic electrical and/or chemical output which, in turn, influences descending systems originating in the midbrain.

1.   Lesion Studies

a.   Medial Preoptic Area. Lesions of the medial preoptic area in female rats are followed by no change in lordosis behavior or by a slight facilitation (Law and Meagher, 1958; Powers and Valenstein, 1972; Singer, 1968). Very small preoptic lesions do not cause any change at all in lordosis in hormone-primed female rats (Raisman and Brown-Grant, 1977) or hamsters (Kow et al., 1974a; Malsbury, Kow, and Pfaff, 1977). Numan (1974) found small increases in lordosis behavior of female rats following either preoptic lesions or bilateral parasagittal knife cuts which would interrupt preoptic axons (Conrad and Pfaff, 1975, 1976a) heading toward the medial forebrain bundle. These lesion results suggest that preoptic neurons have inhibitory effects on lordosis; they are complemented by the electrical stimulation experiments discussed in Section 2.

b.   Suprachiasmatic Nuclei. The suprachiasmatic nuclei help to entrain many biological rhythms with the light cycle, including circadian rhythms of activity and drinking behavior (Stephan and Zucker, 1972a, b), adrenal and pineal rhythms (Muller, 1974), and gonadal function and growth (Rusak and Morin, 1975; Stetson and Watson-Whitmyre, 1976). They are not, however, required for lordosis behavior. Complete destruction of the suprachiasmatic nuclei in female rats (Raisman and Brown-Grant, 1977; Smalstig and Clemens, 1975) or female hamsters (Malsbury et al., 1977) has no effects on lordosis behavior. In cycling ewes, also, suprachiasmatic nucleus lesions have no effect on female reproductive behavior (Domanski, Przekop, and Skubiszewski, 1972). Suprachiasmatic neurons are affected by optic input (Koizumi, Nishino, and Colman, 1975), but suprachiasmatic nucleus cells do not bind estrogen, even though neurons nearby in the medial anterior hypothalamus do accumulate radioactive estradiol (Pfaff, 1968b; Pfaff and Keiner, 1973).

c.   Anterior Hypothalamus. Large lesions of the medial anterior hypothalamus in female rats lead to significant decreases in lordosis, despite treatment with ovarian hormones (Averill and Purves, 1963; Greer, 1953; Herndon and Neill, 1973; Law and Meagher, 1958; Singer, 1968). Small anterior hypothalamic lesions usually are not effective in altering lordosis in female rats (Clark, 1942; Raisman and Brown-Grant, 1977) or hamsters (Malsbury, Kow and Pfaff, 1977). Large lesions at the base of the medial anterior hypothalamus can abolish estrous behavior in female guinea pigs (Brookhart, Dey, and Ranson, 1940, 1941; Dey, 1941; Dey, Fisher, Berry, and Ranson, 1940).

   More selective lesions in female guinea pigs, damaging either the anterior hypothalamic nucleus or the ventromedial nucleus of the hypothalamus, cause a loss of female mating behavior (Goy and Phoenix, 1963). The effects of anterior hypothalamic lesions in female guinea pigs that have been reported were not due to unintended damage of the pituitary, since purposeful lesions of the pituitary did not affect mating behavior (Dey, Leininger, and Ranson, 1942). Similarly, hypophysectomized female rats can respond to estrogen and progesterone injections with normal lordosis behavior (Pfaff, 1970a). In the female cat, also, anterior hypothalamic lesions cause permanent loss of female mating behavior, despite treatment with estrogen (Sawyer, 1960; Sawyer and Robison, 1956). In female cats or rabbits, tuberal lesions lead to losses of mating behavior which can be restored following treatment with exogenous estrogen (Sawyer, 1960; Sawyer and Robison, 1956). Lesions deep in the anterior hypothalamic region of cycling ewes abolishes female mating behavior, and the behavioral loss cannot be ascribed to pituitary or ovarian changes (Clegg, Santolucito, Smith, and Ganong, 1958).

Using coronal transections, Rodgers and Schwartz (1972) studied mating behavior in female rats with intact ovaries. Transections were made at the posterior border of the optic chiasm (i.e., at levels of the anterior hypothalamus just behind the suprachiasmatic nucleus but anterior to the ventromedial nucleus of the hypothalamus). Behavioral testing was done several days after constant vaginal estrus was confirmed. Under these conditions, female rats showed high constant levels of behavioral receptivity. In a similar study, in which the majority of knife cuts were more anterior in the anterior hypothalamus, constant high levels of behavioral receptivity again were shown to accompany persistent vaginal estrus (Rodgers and Schwartz, 1976). To the extent that these cuts actually interrupted anterior hypothalamic fibers which stream through the hypothalamus (Conrad and Pfaff, 1975, 1976b), it can be inferred that lordosis behavior survived a substantial reduction in anterior hypothalamic neuronal influence under conditions of persistent estrus.

Kalra and Sawyer (1970) studied cycling female rats with coronal transections under conditions that made it more difficult to achieve the positive criterion for mating behavior. With anterior hypothalamic transections made on the morning of proestrus, female mating behavior could be shown to be present, under their experimental conditions, only when male rats achieved ejaculation with those females the very night after surgery. These testing conditions served to show the contribution of anterior hypothalamic neurons. With coronal transections at very anterior levels in the hypothalamus (anterior to the suprachiasmatic nuclei), 15 of 18 females mated the night after surgery. However, with transections of posterior borders of the anterior hypothalamus (behind the suprachiasmatic nuclei), only 2 of 10 females mated.

In female hamsters large amounts of damage to anterior hypothalamic cells or fibers disrupts lordosis, even in ovariectomized females primed with estrogen and progesterone (Malsbury et al., 1977; Warner, 1975).

Thus it appears that transections or lesions that remove the influence of a large number of anterior hypothalamic neurons cause a decrease in the performance of lordosis, especially under testing conditions that do not favor appearance of the behavior.

d. Ventromedial Nucleus. Bilateral lesions in and around the ventromedial nucleus of the hypothalamus of the female rat are followed by decreased lordosis performance (Carrer, Asch, Aron, 1973; Dörner, Döcke, and Gotz, 1975; Dörner, Döcke, and Hinz, 1969; Kennedy, 1964; Kennedy and Mitra, 1963; LaVaque and Rodgers, 1974, 1975).

Recently we investigated the effects of electrolytic lesions of the ventromedial nucleus of the hypothalamus on lordosis in ovariectomized female rats. The lesions were made through chronically implanted electrodes. The lesions did not disrupt lordosis immediately, but induced a gradual decline in the reflex (Figure 7–1; Pfaff and Sakuma, 1979a). Lordosis performance reached its minimum no less than 12 hours after the lesion was made and typically after 36–60 hours (Figure 7–2). The magnitude of the behavioral deficit depended on the amount of ventromedial nucleus damage. In fact, on the lateral side of the ventromedial nucleus, lesion size was significantly correlated with lordosis deficit (Pfaff and Sakuma, 1979a). The slow time course of ventromedial lesion and stimulation (Section 2) effects emphasizes the fact that the ventromedial nucleus is not part of a direct reflex arc for lordosis; rather, cells in the ventromedial nucleus exert a tonic hormone-dependent influence on brainstem pathways descending to control this behavior.

In female sheep (Domanski et al., 1972) and female cats (Hagamen and Brooks, 1958) lesions in the region of the ventromedial nucleus abolish behavioral receptivity. Those lesions that have abolished receptivity in female hamsters appear to have been placed at anterior ventromedial levels in such a way that both ventromedial nucleus functions and anterior hypothalamic fibers passing by the ventromedial nucleus would be interrupted (White, 1954). In addition, studies with small lesions

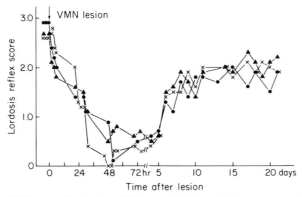

Figure 7–1. Effect on lordosis of bilateral lesion of the ventromedial nucleus (*VMN*) in three representative experiments. Each rat received a daily injection of estrogen throughout the period shown. (From Pfaff & Sakuma, 1979a)

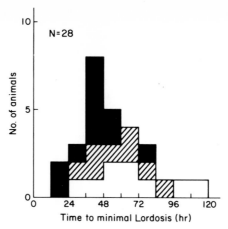

Figure 7–2. Distribution of latencies to the minimal lordosis score following ventromedial hypothalamic lesions. *Black blocks:* animals with severe deficits (lordosis score less than 0.5), *Hatched blocks:* animals with moderate deficits (lordosis less than 1.0). *White blocks:* animals with partial deficits (lordosis less than 1.5). (From Pfaff & Sakuma, 1979a)

confined to the ventromedial nucleus itself show that neurons in this nucleus proper have a primary role in facilitating execution of female reproductive behavior. In female rats, small lesions within the ventromedial nucleus significantly reduce the performance of lordosis during estrogen treatment (Edwards and Mathews, 1977). In female hamsters (Malsbury et al., 1977) the degree of lordosis deficit is significantly correlated with the amount of the ventromedial nucleus destroyed, especially at anterior levels of the ventromedial nucleus (Figure 7–3).

All these results combined lead us to the conclusion that ventromedial nucleus neurons make an important contribution to the execution of lordosis; however, in order to guarantee the abolition of lordosis behavior, lesions should probably disrupt both ventromedial nucleus function and anterior hypothalamic axons that sweep by the ventromedial nucleus.

e.   Summary. Bilateral lesions of the ventromedial nucleus of the hypothalamus and large anterior hypothalamic lesions just anterior to the ventromedial nucleus disrupt the performance of lordosis. The actions of estrogen on these cells relative to female mating behavior, as shown by estrogen binding and the effects of estrogen implants (Chapter 6), lead to the increased cellular activity shown morphologically and electrophysiologically (Chapter 6). Thus, estrogen can facilitate lordosis by acting on the cells that bind it: it increases the biosynthetic and/or electrical activity of these cells, which in turn increases the activity in descending brainstem pathways that facilitate lordosis. Removal of these hypothalamic cells (and therefore of the facilitating estrogen influence) decreases lordosis performance. Conversely, under some conditions, preoptic lesions are followed by increased lordosis performance. Estrogen actions on these cells, demonstrated by estrogen binding and the effects of estrogen implants (Chapter 6), decrease cellular activity as shown by single unit recording (Bueno and Pfaff, 1976). Therefore, estrogen acting to decrease activity in these cells can facilitate lordosis by reducing an influence that is inhibitory to the behavior.

Thus, there are matched differences between medial preoptic neurons and ventromedial hypothalamic neurons both in the physiology of estrogen action and in the sign of their participation in lordosis control. These

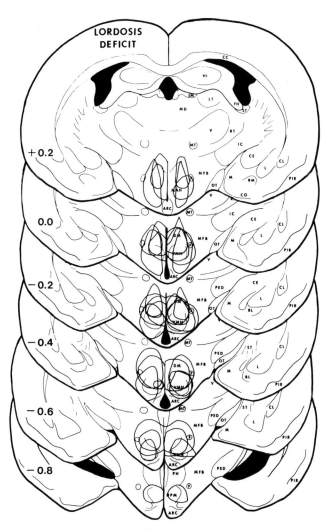

Figure 7-3. Overlapping lesion outlines from the six females with the greatest lordosis deficits. All sustained damage in the region of the ventromedial nucleus. (From Malsbury et al., 1977)

differences tie into a pattern of anatomical and physiological differences between preoptic area–basal forebrain and ventromedial nucleus–posterior hypothalamus. This pattern of differences led to the theory summarized in Section C.

2. Electrical Stimulation

Electrical stimulation of the ventromedial nucleus of the hypothalamus facilitates the lordosis reflex of ovariectomized, estrogen-primed female rats (Pfaff and Sakuma, 1979b). Gradual increases in lordosis performance follow relatively long periods of stimulation. Never less than 15 minutes and usually about 1 hour of electrical stimulation is necessary for maximum facilitation. Following the termination of stimulation, lordosis performance returns gradually to the control level during a 5–8-hour period (Figure 7–4). Optimal frequencies of stimulation are between 10 and 30 Hz (Figure 7–5). Low currents are sufficient; the threshold for effective facilitation averages 12.5 μA. Pretreatment with estrogen is necessary for facilitation by ventromedial nucleus electrical stimulation. The threshold dose for the permissive effect of estrogen is 2.5 μg/rat (Figures 7–6 and 7–7). Electrical stimulation tends to induce larger facilitation when applied to the lateral side of the ventromedial nucleus. Thus, ventromedial nucleus neurons must participate in lordosis control by virtue of a facilitatory output. The delay between the beginning of their stimulation and the beginning of the facilitation effect implies that they are not in the direct reflex arc for lordosis execution; rather, they

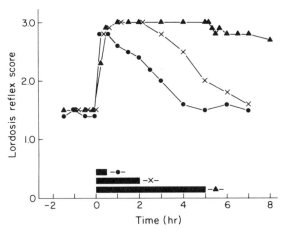

Figure 7–4. Time course of facilitation of lordosis induced by different durations of electrical stimulation of the ventromedial nucleus. Stimulation was given for 0.5, 2, or 5 hours (*black bars*). Stimulus frequency, 10 Hz; 50 μA per electrode; duration of leading (cathodal) pulse, 0.2 milliseconds. (From Pfaff & Sakuma, 1979b)

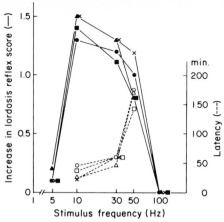

Figure 7–5. Magnitude of increase in lordosis reflex score or latency of facilitation during ventromedial nucleus stimulation at four times threshold intensity in four different animals, as a function of stimulus frequency. (From Pfaff & Sakuma, 1979b)

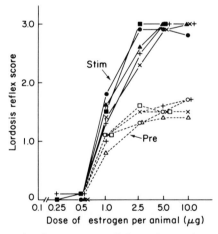

Figure 7–6. Changes in the ventromedial nucleus–stimulated lordosis reflex score *(Stim, solid lines)* or in the prestimulation control score *(Pre, broken lines)* as a function of estradiol benzoate dose. Experiments were done 4 days after estrogen injection. Stimulus parameters were the same as for Figure 7–4, except that the duration was 1 hour. Significant differences ($p < .05$) were seen between control and ventromedial nucleus–stimulated lordosis scores in animals given at least 2.5 μg estradiol benzoate. (From Pfaff & Sakuma, 1979b)

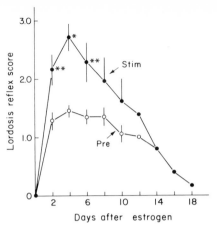

Figure 7–7. Magnitude of the lordosis reflex during ventromedial nucleus electrical stimulation *(Stim, filled circles)* and during prestimulation control periods *(Pre, open circles)* as a function of time after estrogen injection. (Data from Pfaff & Sakuma, 1979b)

must act through a summation or interaction process that has an unusually long time course.

Electrical stimulation of medial preoptic neurons with the same parameters as used for the ventromedial nucleus has the opposite effect: it suppresses the lordosis reflex in female rats (Pfaff and Sakuma, 1979b). Electrical stimulation of the preoptic area in female hamsters also dramatically suppresses lordosis and can interrupt lordosis behavior once started (Figures 7–8 and 7–9; Malsbury, Pfaff, and Malsbury, 1980). This result of preoptic stimulation shows the specificity of the facilitation following stimulation of the ventromedial nucleus. It also shows the opposing roles of preoptic and ventromedial neurons in the control of lordosis.

3. Summary

Neurons in and around the ventromedial nucleus of the hypothalamus facilitate lordosis, whereas medial preoptic neurons suppress it. Partial removal of the ventromedial effect by lesions reduces lordosis perform-

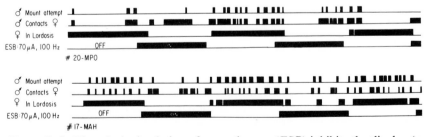

Figure 7–8. Electrical stimulation of preoptic area *(ESB)* inhibits the display (or reinitiation) of lordosis by female hamsters. (From Malsbury et al., 1980)

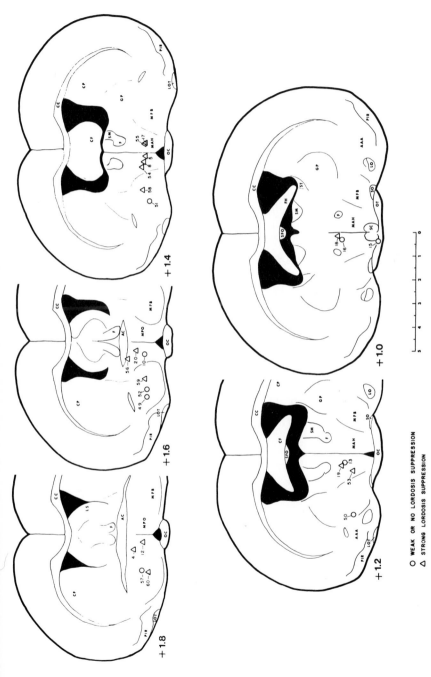

Figure 7–9. Preoptic sites and adjacent locations from which lordosis could be inhibited in female hamsters. (From Malsbury et al. 1980)

ance. Electrical stimulation of ventromedial neurons improves it. In opposition to this influence, electrical stimulation of preoptic neurons suppresses lordosis, whereas preoptic lesions have no effect or increase lordosis performance.

B. Relationship to Control of Ovulation: Luteinizing Hormone–Releasing Hormone (LHRH)

Luteinizing hormone–releasing hormone (LHRH) has been isolated from the hypothalamus, chemically identified, and synthesized (Amoss, Burgus, Blackwell, et al., 1971; Burgus, Butcher, Amoss, et al., 1972; Burgus, Butcher, Ling, et al., 1971; Matsuo, Arimura, Nair, and Schally, 1971; Matsuo, Baba, Nair, et al., 1971; Schally, Baba, Arimura, et al., 1971). Injected systemically, it can cause LH discharge in the female rat pituitary within minutes (Amoss, Blackwell, and Guillemin, 1972; Arimura, Matsuo, Baba, et al., 1972; Monahan, Rivier, Burgus, et al., 1971). During the estrous cycle of the female rat, the ovulatory discharge of LH from the pituitary normally is synchronized with behavioral receptivity, indicated by lordosis (Beach, 1948; Blandau, Boling, and Young, 1941; Feder, Brown-Grant, and Corker, 1971; Schwartz, 1969; Young, Boling, and Blandau, 1941). Therefore, we conducted experiments to see if LHRH could facilitate lordosis in female rats (Pfaff, 1973). We used low doses of estrogen in hypophysectomized, ovariectomized female rats, so that the estrogen alone would not lead to high levels of lordosis behavior. Lower doses of LHRH induced small increases in lordosis behavior, and the higher dose of LHRH led to statistically significant increases (Table 7–1; Pfaff, 1973). LHRH also facilitated lordosis in ovariectomized rats primed with estrone, and control experiments with thyrotropin-releasing factor did not lead to behavioral increases (Moss and McCann, 1973, 1975). Since the female rats in our experiments (Pfaff, 1973) were also hypophysectomized, the lordosis effects of LHRH could not have been due to LH or FSH release; in previous experiments also, these hormones have not proven necessary for steroid-induced behavioral receptivity (Pfaff, 1970a).

Thus, LHRH can facilitate lordosis in the estrogen-primed female rat. This decapeptide both triggers the ovulatory discharge of LH and facilitates a reproductive behavioral response that is closely tied to ovulation during the normal female rat cycle. The behavioral effectiveness of LHRH raises the possibility that some LHRH-producing neurons project to other neurons concerned with lordosis, as well as to the median eminence. Projections to the central gray of the midbrain would be of special interest. Indeed, local microinjections of an antiserum to

Table 7-1. *Effect of LHRH on lordosis behavior in estrogen-primed, hypophysectomized, ovariectomized female rats*

Treatment	No. of rats	Tests positive for lordosis (%)					Lordosis quotient[a] (mean ± SE)				
		Minutes postinjection					Minutes postinjection				
		10	30	90	180	360	10	30	90	180	360
Saline control	20	5	0	8	7	0	6 ± 4	0	5 ± 3	4 ± 3	0
LHRH											
0.4 µg	20	0	0	13	20	15	0	0	10 ± 5	18 ± 7	11 ± 6
4.0 µg	20	0	7	46[b]	57[b]	50[b]	0	4 ± 3	32 ± 6[b]	42 ± 7[b]	34 ± 7[b]

[a](Number of lordoses by female/number of mounts by male) × 100; calculated from results for all tests, including those where the quotients equal zero.

[b]Significantly different from saline controls (*p* < .01).

From Pfaff, 1973b.

Table 7-2. Effects of microinfusion[a] of LHRH or an antibody to LHRH (anti-LHRH G) on lordosis behavior[b] in an ovariectomized estrogen-treated female rat

Substance infused	Preinfusion control	Minutes postinfusion							
		5	10	15	30	60	120	180	720
LHRH	1.5	2.1	2.8	2.9	2.9	2.8	1.2	0	0
anti-LHRH G	1.7	1.0	0.9	0.6	0.4	0	0	0.2	0.4

[a]Site of microinfusion was midbrain central gray.

[b]Maximum lordosis amplitude is 3.0.

Data from Sakuma & Pfaff 1980a.

LHRH applied to the central gray of the midbrain can block lordosis behavior (Table 7–2; Sakuma and Pfaff, 1980a). Therefore, projections from the hypothalamus carrying LHRH to the central gray of the midbrain may be important for the control of lordosis behavior. In fact, the time required for LHRH synthesis, transport, and use may account for the slow actions of hypothalamic cells on lordosis behavior referred to above.

C.   Relationship of Female Behavior to Male Behavior and Autonomic Control Mechanisms: A Theory

1.   Female Reproductive Function

The net effect of medial preoptic tissue on lordosis is a decrease in performance of the reflex, while the net effect of hypothalamic tissue in and around the ventromedial nucleus is facilitation of lordosis (see above). Studies in the control of ovulation also show differing roles for the medial preoptic area and basomedial hypothalamus in female rats. Basomedial hypothalamic tissue is sufficient for tonic gonadotropin release and negative feedback effects of steroids in female rats, whereas the medial preoptic area is required for normal ovulation and cyclicity (Barraclough and Gorski, 1961; Halasz, 1969; Halasz and Gorski, 1967). Electrochemical stimulation of the preoptic area and of basal forebrain tissue anterior to the preoptic area (diagonal bands of Broca and septum) can stimulate ovulatory surges of LH release in female rats (Everett, 1969; Kubo, Mennin, and Gorski, 1975); the mechanism of this effect is being investigated with electrophysiological techniques (Dyer and Burnet, 1976; Terasawa and Sawyer, 1969). Recording of preoptic area multiple unit activity (Kawakami et al., 1970) and single unit activity (Wuttke, 1974) has shown a correlation between increased preoptic neuronal firing rate and increased release of LH. In the control of growth hormone also, preoptic oppose basomedial hypothalamic influences: preoptic neurons decrease growth hormone secretion, whereas ventro-medial hypothalamic neurons increase it (Martin, 1979).

Regarding the control of lordosis, certain areas of the basal forebrain share with the medial preoptic area the function of suppressing female reproductive behavior. Large lesions of the lateral septum are followed by impressive increases in the lordosis performance of estrogen-primed female rats (Nance, Shryne, and Gorski, 1974, 1975). Conversely, elec-trical stimulation of the septal area suppresses lordosis (Zasorin, Mals-bury, and Pfaff, 1975). Control lesions in the amygdala have neither facilitating nor suppressing effects on lordosis (Nance et al., 1974), but amygdala destruction may interact with the septal effect (Nance, Mc-Ginnis, and Gorski, 1976). Basal forebrain suppression of lordosis may be related to olfactory function, since olfactory ablations are followed by increased lordosis performance in hormone-primed female rats (Ed-wards and Warner, 1972; Moss, 1971; Nance et al., 1976). Lordosis suppression by the basal forebrain may operate by input to the preoptic area (Yamanouchi and Arai, 1975) or by effects on a common neural substrate farther downstream in lordosis circuits. In any case, medial preoptic and lateral septal neurons seem to share a role in the suppression of lordosis, and their effect is opposite to the effect of the basomedial hypothalamus.

Estrogen from the circulation has a suppressive effect on the single unit activity of neurons in the medial preoptic area as shown by records of spontaneous activity and responsivity to peripheral stimuli (Bueno and Pfaff, 1976; Lincoln, 1967; Whitehead and Ruf, 1974; Yagi, 1970, 1973). In contrast, estrogen increases the single unit activity of hypothalamic tissue posterior to the preoptic area, especially in the basomedial hypo-thalamus (Bueno and Pfaff, 1976; Cross and Dyer, 1972; Kawakami, Terasawa, Ibuki, and Manaka, 1971). It should also be noted that neurochemical effects of estrogen on enzyme activities are not the same in the preoptic area as they are in the basomedial hypothalamus (Luine, Khylchevskaya, and McEwen, 1974, 1975a,b). In addition, Brawer and Sonnenschein (1975) showed effects of estrogen on fine structure in arcuate neurons without such effects showing up in the medial preoptic area, and Araki, Ferin, Zimmerman, and Vande Wiele, (1975) showed different effects of ovariectomy on LRF content in basomedial as opposed to far anterior hypothalamic tissue.

Thus, with respect to lordosis control, ovulation control, and the electrophysiological and neurochemical effects of estrogen, there is a clear bifurcation of function between the medial preoptic area (along with the basal forebrain) and the basomedial hypothalamus.

2.   Male Mating Behavior

Medial preoptic neurons stimulate masculine mating behavior and are required for its normal performance (reviewed by Malsbury and Pfaff, 1974). Electrical stimulation of the medial preoptic area of male rats facilitates various aspects of male copulatory behavior (Malsbury, 1971). Similar data have been gathered from other species. Electrical stimulation of the medial preoptic area of male opossums triggers mounting and other male mating responses (Roberts, Steinberg, and Means, 1967), and similar data have been gathered using the male guinea pig (Martin, 1976). At least part of the facilitatory influence of the preoptic area on male mating behavior must be due to the effects of testosterone (or testosterone metabolites) on preoptic neurons. Autoradiographic experiments have shown that testosterone is strongly accumulated by preoptic neurons (Pfaff, 1968a). Single unit recording from preoptic cells has shown that systemic injections of testosterone or direct application of testosterone to the preoptic region in anesthetized castrated male rats can alter spontaneous discharge rates and responsivity to peripheral stimuli by preoptic neurons (Pfaff and Pfaffmann, 1969). Indeed, implantation of testosterone into the preoptic area of adult (Davidson, 1966; Johnston and Davidson, 1972; Lisk, 1967) and neonatal (Christensen and Gorski, 1976) rats significantly facilitates masculine reproductive behavior, and they can restore male sex behavior in castrated male rats.

Preoptic facilitation is required for male mating behavior, since many studies have shown that medial preoptic lesions can reduce or abolish sex behavior in male animals (references in Malsbury and Pfaff, 1974). The importance of the medial preoptic area for masculine mating behavior is not restricted to male rodents; medial preoptic neurons have been strongly implicated in the control of male sex behavior in a wide variety of mammals, birds, amphibia, and fish (Kelley and Pfaff, 1978).

Axons of preoptic neurons important for male sex behavior leave the preoptic area running laterally toward the medial forebrain bundle. Parasagittal knife cuts separating the medial preoptic area from the medial forebrain bundle severely impair male sex behavior (Paxinos, 1973; Paxinos and Bindra, 1972; Szechtman, Caggiula, and Wulkan, 1975). Coronal transections behind the preoptic area in the medial hypothalamus (Paxinos and Bindra, 1972) and transections that spare preoptic tissue near the base of the brain (Rodgers, 1969) do not significantly affect male mating responses, showing that the critical axons run laterally, not posteriorly through the medial hypothalamus, and that some critical axons run near the bottom of the brain. These results suggest that axons of neurons important for male sex behavior travel posteriorly in the medial forebrain bundle; this interpretation can predict results of medial forebrain bundle lesions and electrical stimulation.

As expected, medial forebrain bundle lesions disrupt or abolish masculine mating responses by male rats (Caggiula, Antelman, and Zigmond,

1973; Caggiula, Gay, Antelman, and Leggens, 1975; Hitt, Bryon, and Modianos, 1973; Hitt, Hendricks, Ginsberg, and Lewis, 1970; Modianos, Flexman, and Hitt, 1973). The same type of medial forebrain bundle lesions do not disrupt female reproductive behavior (Hitt et al., 1970; Modianos et al., 1973); in fact, under some endocrine conditions, medial forebrain bundle lesions can lead to an elevation of lordosis performance, similar to the effect seen with preoptic area lesions (Modianos, Delia, and Pfaff, 1976). Masculine mating behavior is facilitated by electrical stimulation of the medial forebrain bundle (Caggiula, 1970; Caggiula and Hoebel, 1966; Eibergen and Caggiula, 1973). All of these results are consistent with the idea that medial preoptic neurons sending their axons posteriorly through the medial forebrain bundle are essential for the facilitation of male, but not female reproductive behavior.

Neuroanatomical findings support the inferences from lesion and electrical stimulation studies. Medial preoptic neurons (in the preoptic regions governing male mating behavior) have been shown to send their axons through the medial portions of the medial forebrain bundle, while medial anterior hypothalamic and ventromedial nucleus neurons (in the regions essential for female mating behavior) do not send descending axons through the medial forebrain bundle (Conrad and Pfaff, 1975, 1976a,b). Whereas neurons from the ventromedial nucleus of the hypothalamus and medial anterior hypothalamus project strongly to the dorsal (as well as ventral) central gray of the mesencephalon and to the lateral midbrain reticular formation of the mesencephalon, medial preoptic neurons do not have these strong projections. Furthermore, preoptic neurons and medial basal hypothalamic neurons differ in their patterns of projection to the lateral septal nucleus.

Differences in the strength and nature of synaptic effects (Mancia, 1974) as well as site of terminations could underlie differences between preoptic–basal forebrain functions and basomedial–posterior hypothalamic functions. However, the axonal projections demonstrated thus far provide possible anatomical substrates for separate neural systems mediating male and female sex behaviors: preoptic neurons projecting through the medial forebrain bundle, critical for male mating responses, and basomedial hypothalamic neurons projecting to the mesencephalic central gray and lateral reticular formation, critical for female mating responses.

3. Autonomic Function

Hess (1954, 1957) electrically stimulated the brains of freely moving cats and observed autonomic effects. Electrical stimulation of the preoptic area, medial thalamus, and basal forebrain (notably the septum) was followed by decreased blood pressure, decreased heart rate, decreased

respiratory activity, pupillary constriction, and the initiation of micturi-
tion, defecation, and salivation. Electrical stimulation of the posterior
hypothalamus and the periventricular system leading to the central gray
matter of the mesencephalon was followed by increased blood pressure,
increased heart rate, increased respiratory activity, and pupillary dilata-
tion. Based on these observations, we proposed that the preoptic area
and basal forebrain primarily serve a parasympathetic or antisympathetic
function ("trophotropic" function) and the posterior hypothalamus primarily serves a sympathetic ("ergotropic") function.

Modern work has borne out Hess' experimental observations. Electrical stimulation of the preoptic region and basal forebrain (especially
the septum) consistently yields decreases in blood pressure and heart
rate (Ahmed, 1974; Brickman, Calaresu, and Mogenson, 1979; Ciriello,
Calaresu, and Mogenson, 1975; Hilton and Spyer, 1971; Takeuchi and
Manning, 1973; Zehr, 1973). Electrical stimulation of the basomedial
hypothalamus (including the ventromedial and dorsomedial nuclei) and
the posterior hypothalamus reliably elicit increases in blood pressure and
heart rate (Ahmed, 1974; Bagshaw, Iizuka, and Peterson, 1971; Calaresu,
1974; Djojosugito, Folkow, Kylstra, et al., 1970; Takeuchi and Manning,
1973; Verrier, Calvert, and Lown, 1975).

Association of the preoptic area with parasympathetic (or antisympathetic) functions may explain two types of observations reported after
preoptic lesions. First, in the preoptic lesion and transection experiments
in which male mating behavior was reduced or abolished (references
above), some authors reported that the lesioned males mounted the
female, but intromissions were not achieved. In any case where intromission was achieved, it was reported that several could then be achieved
by the same animal and ejaculation resulted. These qualitative observations are consistent with the notion that the main failure in male mating
behavior after preoptic lesions is the inability to achieve an intromission,
and that in turn could be explained by the inability to have an erection.
Since erection requires parasympathetic activity (or inhibition of sympathetic function), the failure of intromission (or erection) could be
described as a failure of parasympathetic function. This is consistent
with the findings concerning the role of the preoptic area in autonomic
physiology (reviewed above). Thus, the importance of preoptic neurons
for parasympathetic (or antisympathetic) functions provides a mechanism
for the participation of the preoptic region in male mating behavior: these
neurons are required to allow the male to achieve an erection, and thus
an intromission.

A second type of observation following preoptic lesions, usually an
unintentional effect, is the death of the experimental animal due to
pulmonary edema. Pulmonary edema results from abnormally intense
systemic vasoconstriction (Chen and Chai, 1974). It can thus be described
as a failure of antisympathetic functions, which, according to the results
reviewed above, is the expected result after preoptic lesions. Preoptic

lesions would allow abnormally high systemic vasoconstriction, which in turn would result in abnormally high central blood pressures, leading to pulmonary edema. Thus, both intended and unintended results of preoptic lesion studies on male mating behavior can be explained by the parasympathetic role of preoptic tissue.

Association of the basomedial and posterior hypothalamus with sympathetic autonomic functions and female reproductive behavior may underlie the muscular activity required for the increased locomotion shown by the estrous female rat.

4.   Theory

The comparison of medial preoptic (and basal forebrain) tissue with basomedial (and posterior) hypothalamus is summarized in Table 7–3 and presented schematically in Figure 7–10. Briefly, preoptic neurons are required for male mating behavior but suppress female mating behavior. They have a parasympathetic (or antisympathetic) function. The types of effects estradiol has on these neurons are consistent with their role in female mating behavior. The association of preoptic tissue with parasympathetic function provides an explanation of the mechanism of preoptic control over male mating behavior and also explains deaths due to pulmonary edema following preoptic lesions. It appears (Chapter 8) that preoptic neurons exert descending influences through axons that travel in the medial part of the medial forebrain bundle.

Basomedial hypothalamic neurons are not required for male mating behavior but are required for normal female mating behavior. Effects of estrogen on these neurons are consistent with their role in governing female reproductive behavior responses. Basomedial and posterior hypothalamic neurons serve a sympathetic autonomic function. This may support the greatly increased running activity shown by the receptive female rat under the influence of estrogen. Axons descending from basomedial hypothalamic neurons do not travel in the medial forebrain bundle (Chapter 8). Strong projections from these neurons to the midbrain central gray matter and the lateral portions of the midbrain reticular formation may be important for mediating descending influences from the basomedial and posterior hypothalamus.

D.   Source and Sign of Net Hypothalamic Influence on Lordosis Behavior

Decerebrate female rats do not perform lordosis behavior (Kow et al., 1978). Following complete transections of the brainstem between the colliculi or at the diencephalic–mesencephalic junction, ovariectomized

Table 7-3. *Comparison of medial preoptic area (and basal forebrain) with basomedial (and posterior) hypothalamus: Brief summary of some major differences*

Parameter	Medial preoptic area[a]	Basomedial hypothalamus[a]
Reproductive function		
Male mating behavior	↑	0
Female mating behavior	↓	↑
Effect on LH	Ovulation surge (positive feedback)	Negative feedback
Effect of estradiol on unit activity	↓	↑
Autonomic function		
Blood pressure	↓	↑
Heart rate	↓	↑
Diameter of pupil	↓	↑
Micturition, defecation, salivation	↑	
Anatomical projections		
Descending axon trajectories	MFB	Outside MFB
To midbrain central gray	Weak	Strong
To lateral midbrain reticular formation	Weak	Strong
To lateral septum	Dorsal	Midlateral

[a] ↑, increases; ↓, decreases; 0, no effect; MFB, medial forebrain bundle.
From Pfaff & Modianos, 1980.

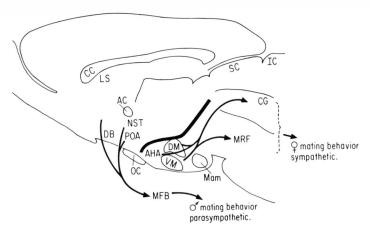

Figure 7–10. Summary of theoretical division of preoptic and hypothalamic tissue, according to its participation in the control of male or female mating behavior in rats. This division may correspond to the differential participation of preoptic and basomedial (and posterior) hypothalamic tissue in the control of sympathetic and parasympathetic autonomic nervous system functions. In the case of male mating behavior, there are likely causal relationships with preoptic tissue participation in parasympathetic functions. (From Pfaff & Modianos, 1980) *Abbreviations: AC,* anterior commissure; *AHA,* anterior hypothalamic area; *CC,* corpus callosum; *CG,* central gray; *DB,* diagonal bands; *DM,* dorsomedial nucleus of hypothalamus; *IC,* inferior colliculus; *LS,* lateral septal nucleus; *Mam,* mammillary bodies; *MFB,* medial forebrain bundle; *MRF,* mesencephalic reticular formation; *NST,* bed nucleus of stria terminalis; *OC,* optic chiasm; *POA,* preoptic area; *SC,* superior colliculus; *VM,* ventromedial nucleus of hypothalamus.

female rats treated with estrogen and progesterone were tested for lordosis behavior as well as other physiological parameters (Figure 7–11). Lordosis disappeared after decerebration but not after control operations.

These results indicate that a net facilitatory influence from the telencephalon or diencephalon is required for lordosis to occur. An obvious source of this facilitatory influence is the ventromedial nucleus of the hypothalamus, since lesions there disrupt lordosis (Section A). In fact, the source of the lordosis-facilitating influence must be neurons in and around the ventromedial hypothalamic nucleus, because of all other diencephalic and telencephalic forebrain tissue with projections to the midbrain, there are no other potential sources in which lesions lead to a loss of lordosis.

Let us consider first the forebrain tissue outside the limbic system and hypothalamus. The cerebral cortex is not required for lordosis, and, in fact, cortical loss can actually improve lordosis behavior (Beach, 1944; Clemens, Wallen, and Gorski, 1967). Similarly, thalamic tissue can be eliminated from consideration, partly because its main job is to communicate with the cerebral cortex (which is unnecessary for lordosis), and

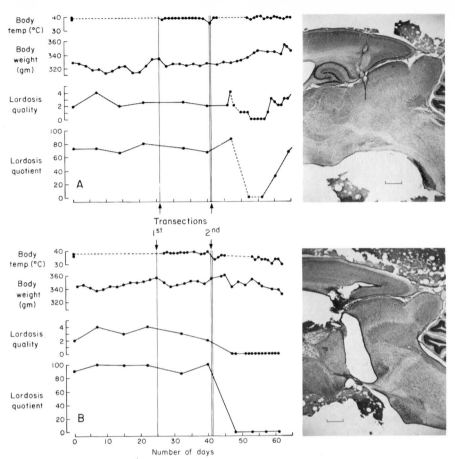

Figure 7–11 A and B. Results before and after brain transections, each made in two stages (first one side, then the other). (A) Rat with control, shallow transection. (B) Rat with complete brainstem transection, producing a chronic decerebrate female rat. *Left-hand side:* experimental results *Broken lines* in the body temperature curves: temperature was not taken. *Broken lines* in lordosis quality and lordosis quotient of control animal: the period that ovarian hormones were not given. The data for the control rat are not shown beyond Day 65, after which the control rat was given rat chow and water ad libitum instead of tube feeding. The temperature and body weight remained constant and both lordosis quality and quotient remained high until the rat was sacrificed. *Right-hand side:* photomicrographs showing the extent of transections. The calibration is 1 mm. (From Kow et al., 1978)

partly because large bilateral transections can be made through the thalamus without an effect on lordosis (Manogue et al., 1980a). Finally, olfactory input and the olfactory bulbs and system are not required for lordosis, since olfactory ablations are followed by no change or increased lordosis performance (Edwards and Warner, 1972; Kow and Pfaff, 1976; Moss, 1971; Nance et al., 1976).

Considering limbic tissue, the amygdala is not required for lordosis (Nance et al., 1974, 1976). Abolition of the main output of the amygdala in the rat, the stria terminalis, has no effect on female reproductive function (Raisman and Brown-Grant, 1977). Large lesions of the hippocampus have no effect on lordosis behavior (Kimble, Rogers, and Hendrickon, 1967), and lesions of the septum actually improve lordosis (Nance et al., 1974, 1975).

As documented above, no hypothalamic tissue other than those cells in and around the ventromedial nucleus is required for lordosis. Similarly, cells with axons in the medial forebrain bundle (whether they be hypothalamic cells or other cells in the forebrain) are not required for lordosis, since large lesions of the medial forebrain bundle in some cases have no effect on lordosis and in other cases allow for slight improvement of lordosis (Modianos et al., 1976).

Therefore, considering all lesion studies treating forebrain tissue in the diencephalon or telencephalon, no tissue other than the ventromedial nucleus of the hypothalamus has been shown to be important for the facilitation of lordosis. Thus, the net facilitatory influence of the forebrain on lordosis behavior must come from cells in and around the ventromedial hypothalamic nucleus.

E.   Summary

Cells in and around the ventromedial nucleus of the hypothalamus facilitate lordosis. Lesions of these cells lead to loss of lordosis. Electrical stimulation of these cells at low frequencies leads to lordosis facilitation. No other lesion or electrical stimulation sites in the forebrain can account for the facilitation of lordosis behavior by forebrain tissue. Therefore, among all telencephalic and diencephalic sites, the main source of lordosis facilitation must be the cells in and around the ventromedial hypothalamic nucleus (Figure 6–10).

Luteinizing hormone releasing hormone (LHRH) facilitates lordosis behavior in ovariectomized hypophysectomized female rats. This effect may provide the slow mechanism by which hypothalamic cells act on the midbrain to promote female reproductive behavior.

Through their control of both male and female reproductive behavior, hypothalamic cells link behavioral mechanisms to autonomic controls and endocrine rhythms. Thus, in this way, they integrate behavioral responses with other aspects of the physiology of the organism.

Chapter 8
Hypothalamic Outflow

A. Introduction

We have known for decades that the hypothalamus participates in the control of essential behavioral, endocrine, and autonomic functions. Interference with hypothalamic cell groups can disrupt food intake, drinking, temperature regulation, aggressive behavior, emotional responses, maternal functions, sleep, arousal, secretion of hormones from the pituitary, and reproductive beahvior. Regarding lordosis, hypothalamic axons descending to the midbrain provide an obligatory facilitation (Kow et al., 1978). Moreover, axons exiting the hypothalamus presumably carry the signals that differentiate male and female behavioral functions and integrate behavioral responses with autonomic changes.

The great functional importance of the hypothalamus has been proven by a wealth of behavioral, physiological, and endocrine studies. However, until recently, very few anatomical studies were available to suggest which hypothalamic projections to other brain regions might effect behavioral changes. The lack of neuroanatomical data on hypothalamic projections resulted mainly from technical difficulties in using the classical neuroanatomical tracing methods with hypothalamic cells (for a more complete discussion, see Conrad and Pfaff, 1976a). Hypothalamic and preoptic axons are of very fine caliber, and thus are difficult to stain with reduced silver methods (Valverde, 1965; Sutin, 1966; Chi, 1970). Fibers of passage through the preoptic area and hypothalamus also make it difficult to study the projections of hypothalamic and preoptic cell bodies using anatomical techniques that rely on lesions. Finally, Golgi studies (Valverde, 1965) had indicated that preoptic and hypothalamic neurons have no long axon projections.

With the advent of tritiated amino acid autoradiography (Cowan, Gottelieb, Hendrickson, et al., 1972; Hendrickson, 1975) as an anatomical technique for tracing neuronal projections, studies with hypothalamic and preoptic neurons became more practical. The tritiated amino acid autoradiographic method, as we have used it, circumvents the problems inherent in confusing projections from nerve cell bodies with those from fibers of passage: tritiated amino acids injected or iontophoresed directly in the neighborhood of the cell bodies to be studied are taken up and incorporated into proteins by the cell bodies. These radioactively labeled proteins are then transported by axoplasmic flow from the cell body down the axon and into the axon terminals. Axons passing by the cell bodies in question do not contain protein-synthetizing structures, and thus do not incorporate and transport the isotope. Furthermore, even the smallest axons show these phenomena, and the reduced silver grains in the autoradiogram are always visible. Thus, this method is sensitive, even for axons of very fine caliber. Sensitivity is further increased simply by lengthening the exposure time for the autoradiograms (Conrad and Pfaff, 1975, 1976a).

We have determined the patterns of axonal projections from neurons in cell groups in the medial hypothalamus and preoptic area. Our purpose was partly to complete the neuronal circuit for lordosis behavior, and, more generally, to lay an anatomical foundation for electrophysiological studies of the hypothalamus.

B.   Preoptic Area

Charts from tritiated amino acid autoradiograms showing the full pattern of axonal projections from a typical group of medial preoptic cells are presented in Figure 8–1. Projections from neighboring sites within and near the medial preoptic area (for instance, the periventricular preoptic area and the bed nucleus of the stria terminalis) have also been illustrated (Conrad and Pfaff, 1976a).

Axons taveling anterior from the cell bodies labeled as shown in Figure 8–1 travel through the diagonal end of Broca. Some continue dorsally with the diagonal bands into the septum, terminating in the ventral, dorsal, and anterior septal nuclei, but leaving a diagonally oval region in the midlateral septum relatively free of label.

Other preoptic axons turn dorsally from the injection site into the stria medullaris, stria terminalis, or periventricular thalamus. Labeled fibers in the stria medullaris travel caudally into the lateral habenula. Those in the stria terminalis terminate in the medial amygdala. Other preoptic projections to the medial amygdala pass directly laterally from the labeled cell bodies and reach the amygdala by coursing through the substantia innominata or just above the optic tract.

Many preoptic axons turn caudally from the injection site to descend in the medial forebrain bundle. Descending preoptic fibers in the medial forebrain bundle are clumped in the medial portion of this tract, just

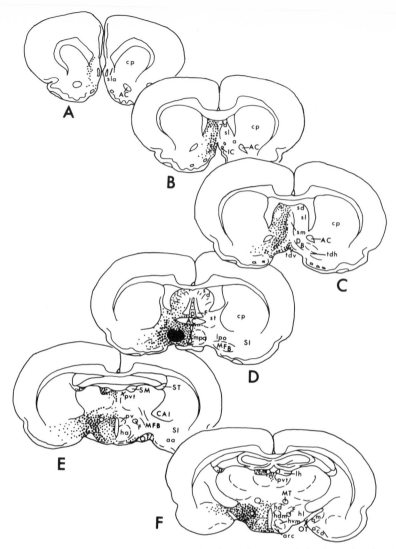

Figure 8–1. Distribution of labeled projections from an injection site in the medial preoptic area. *Large black dots:* labeled fibers. *Small black dots:* fields of individual grains. *Solid black area:* region of labeled cell bodies (injection site). (From Congrad & Pfaff, 1976a)

lateral to the fornix. Some of these descending axons turn medially from the medial forebrain bundle and are traced into the internal layer of the median eminence or the arcuate nucleus. Within the medial hypothalamus, the paraventricular nucleus, dorsomedial nucleus, and ventrolateral subdivision of the ventromedial nucleus receive projections from medial preoptic cells.

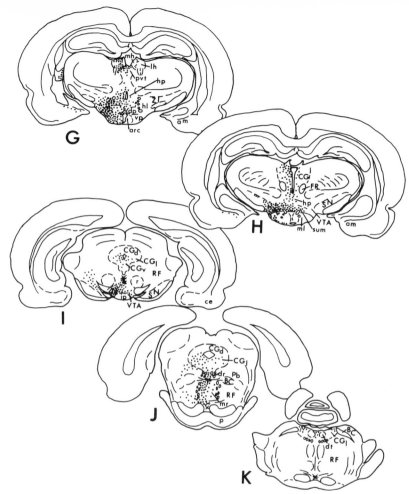

Figure 8–1. (Continued)

At premammillary levels, most preoptic axons remain clumped in the medial forebrain bundle just lateral to the mammillothalamic tract and fornix. Some preoptic axons turn medially to distribute in the ventral premammillary and supramammillary nuclei. Other fibers branch dorso-medially into the periventricular fiber system headed for the central gray. In the midbrain, the midlateral, medial, and ventral central gray receive light bilateral projections from the medial preoptic area. No labeled fibers can be followed into the dorsal region of the midbrain central gray.

No preoptic projections are found in the mammillary bodies, although some labeled axons course through them on their way to the ventral tegmental area. In the ventral tegmental area, preoptic axons that had remained ventral become scattered and diffuse. Some labeled fibers turn dorsally to distribute in the median and dorsal raphe nuclei. Others curve laterally, beneath the medial lemniscus, to reach the midbrain reticular formation. Preoptic projections to the reticular formation do not extend into the pons. The most posterior projection observed from the medial preoptic area reaches the pontine central gray just anterior to the locus coeruleus (Conrad and Pfaff, 1976a).

Axons from preoptic cell bodies still more medial, in the periventricular strata, have a distribution similar to those just described, but their longest axoned projections are weaker. Periventricular preoptic neurons do not send axons through the stria medullaris but do project more heavily than other preoptic cell groups to the arcuate nucleus and median eminence.

For comparison, projections from neurons in the bed nucleus of the stria terminalis were also studied. In most respects they are similar to those from the medial preoptic area, with the addition of a projection to the accessory olfactory bulb. Their axons within the medial forebrain bundle tend to run dorsally to those from medial preoptic neurons.

In contrast, neurons in the nuclei of the diagnonal band of Broca show a much different pattern of axonal projections from the medial preoptic area, the bed nucleus of the stria terminalis, or (see below) the medial anterior hypothalamus (Table 8-1). For instance, these neurons project to the medial septum and the hippocampus. Axons descending from cells in the nuclei of the diagonal band of Broca run in the ventral portion of the medial forebrain bundle. There are hardly any projections from these neurons to the medial hypothalamus, but the medial mammillary nuclei (which do not receive preoptic projections) do receive axons from the nuclei of the diagonal bands. Axons from diagonal band nuclei run to the medial as well as the lateral habenula, and also are found in the mediodorsal thalamic nucleus.

Table 8-1. Summary of projections from the nuclei in the diagonal band of Broca (NDB), vs. medial preoptic area (MPOA), and anterior hypothalamic area (AHA)

Brain region receiving projection	NDB	MPOA and AHA
Amygdala	Basolateral	Medial
Hippocampus	Yes	No
Thalamus	Mediodorsal	Periventricular
Habenula	Medial and lateral	Lateral
Medial hypothalamus	No	Yes
Mammillary bodies	Medial	Fibers through
Central gray	No	Yes
Midbrain reticular formation	No	Yes

From Pfaff & Conrad, 1978.

C. Medial Anterior Hypothalamus

Charts from tritiated amino acid autoradiograms showing the full pattern of axonal projections from a typical cell group in the medial anterior hypothalamus are presented in Figure 8–2. Projections from other cell groups within and near the medial anterior hypothalamus (for instance, the periventricular anterior hypothalamus and the paraventricular nucleus) have also been illustrated (Conrad and Pfaff, 1976b).

Labeled axons ascending from anterior hypothalamic cells cross through the preoptic area to join the diagonal band of Broca. The bed nuclei of the stria terminalis and of the diagonal band receive projections. From the diagonal band, anterior hypothalamic axons turn to distribute in the septum. A diagonally oval region in the midlateral septum becomes especially heavily labeled (this is the same septal region left unlabeled by medial preoptic neurons).

From the anterior hypothalamus, other labeled axons travel dorsally into the stria medullaris, stria terminalis, and midline thalamus. Anterior hypothalamic axons in the stria medullaris distribute in the lateral habenula, while those in the stria terminalis reach the medial amygdala. Axons also reach the medial amygdala by coursing directly laterally from the injection site, and by running laterally in the supraoptic commissure above the optic tract.

Many anterior hypothalamic axons descend to more posterior brain regions. These axons do not run in the medial forebrain bundle; rather, they descend through the hypothalamus proper, in a bundle ventromedial to the fornix.

From this bundle of axons, a few labeled fibers turn medially, crossing in the supraoptic commissure to distribute in the contralateral hypothalamus. Other anterior hypothalamic axons enter the internal layer of the median eminence and the arcuate nucleus. Within the hypothalamus, strong projections enter the dorsomedial nucleus and all subdivisions of the ventromedial nucleus.

Just caudal to the ventromedial nucleus, many anterior hypothalamic axons descending in the bundle ventromedial to the fornix begin to curve dorsomedially. These fibers continue dorsally and caudally into the periventricular fiber system and central gray. Others scatter medial to the fornix in a heavy projection to the dorsal premammillary nucleus. Still others distribute to the supramammillary nucleus and course around or through the mammillary nuclei to reach the ventral tegmental area. From there, some axons turn laterally to reach the midbrain reticular formation. A few spread dorsally into the median and dorsal raphe nuclei.

Anterior hypothalamic axons that had swept dorsally into the rostral midbrain central gray give rise to a very strong projection within the central gray, covering all central gray subdivisions except a dorsolateral

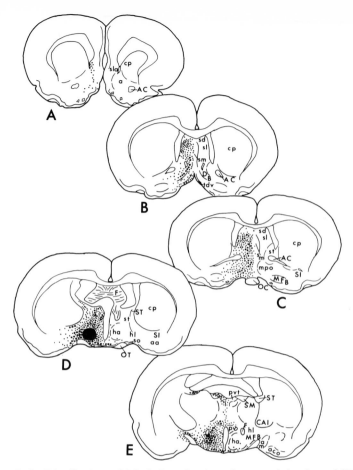

Figure 8–2. Distribution of labeled projections from an injection of ³H-proline into the mid- and perifornical regions of the medial anterior hypothalamus (transverse sections). Symbols as in Figure 8–1. (From Conrad & Pfaff, 1976b)

corner and the most ventral portion. Some labeled axons even spread dorsally through the posterior commissure or laterally into the midbrain reticular formation. The most posterior projections from the anterior hypothalamus extend to the lateral pontine central gray immediately anterior to the locus ceruleus (Conrad and Pfaff, 1976b).

For comparison, projections from the paraventricular nucleus were also studied (Conrad and Pfaff, 1976b). Projections from paraventricular neurons are not restricted to the median eminence and posterior pituitary. In the brain, they distribute to many of the same regions as those covered by anterior hypothalamic neurons, but have somewhat different trajectories and longer descending projections. For instance, we found paraventricular neuron projections to the nucleus of the tractus solitarius in the medulla, and saw some fibers heading into the spinal cord.

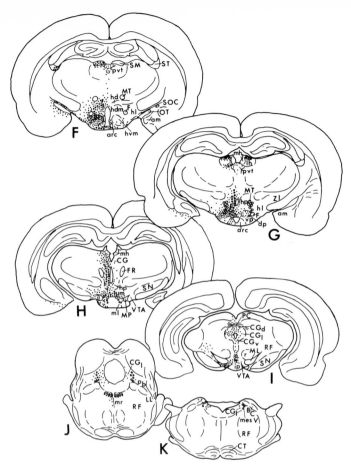

Figure 8–2. (Continued)

Projections from anterior hypothalamic cells are distinct from those of the medial preoptic area (Table 8-2). For example, whereas anterior

Table 8-2. Summary of projections from the medial preoptic area (MPOA) **vs.** *medial anterior hypothalamic area (MAHA)*

Brain region receiving projection	MPOA	MAHA
Septum	Dorsal	Midlateral
Axons in medial forebrain bundle	Yes	No
Axons ventromedial to fornix	No	Yes
Ventromedial nucleus	Ventrolateral	All subdivisions
Premammillary nuclei	Ventral	Dorsal
Midbrain central gray	Ventral	Dorsal and ventral

From Pfaff & Conrad, 1978.

hypothalamic axons descend in a bundle ventromedial to the fornix, medial preoptic axons run in the medial forebrain bundle. Importantly, anterior hypothalamic axons give rise to a strong projection to the dorsal as well as middle central gray, while preoptic projections are restricted to a relatively weak distribution in the ventral central gray. Altogether, these differences in anatomical projections may underlie the functional differences between the medial preoptic area and the anterior hypothalamus, for instance their different participation in the control of male and female sex behavior.

D. Ventromedial Nucleus of the Hypothalamus

Charts of tritiated amino acid autoradiograms showing the full pattern of axonal projections from the ventromedial nucleus of the hypothalamus are presented in Figure 8–3. Projections from other injection sites (for instance, from the anterior, ventrolateral, and dorsomedial portions of the ventromedial nucleus, and just posterior to the ventromedial nucleus) also have been illustrated (Krieger, Conrad, and Pfaff, 1979). Of all the hypothalamic projection patterns described in this chapter, axons descending from the ventromedial nucleus are likely to be the most important for the control of lordosis behavior.

Some axons ascend from the ventromedial nucleus through the anterior hypothalamus at its ventral border, while others rise dorsally. Among the ventral ascending fibers, some follow the route of the tuberoinfundibular tract medially, while others travel lateral to the suprachiasmatic nucleus. The more dorsal ascending axons result in projections to the periventricular thalamus and the bed nucleus of the stria terminalis. Labeled axons reach the lateral septum, with the heaviest projections in the ventralateral portion.

Axons heading laterally from the ventromedial nucleus are prominent. Those heading anterolaterally fan across the medial forebrain bundle. Some penetrate the cerebral peduncle, and many reach as far as the anterior amygdaloid area.

At caudal levels of the ventromedial nucleus, two groups of fibers travel laterally. One heads dorsolaterally, dorsal to the cerebral peduncle, through the fields of Forel and the zona incerta. The other heads more ventrally and enters the ventral supraoptic commissure. Although many of the fibers entering the supraoptic commissure appear to contribute to the descending projection to the mesencephalon, some clearly terminate in the amygdala, primarily in the medial and a specific portion of the cortical amygdaloid nuclei.

Most interesting from the point of view of reproductive behavior control, many lateral-going ventromedial nucleus axons continue descending, curving lateral and dorsal as they go. Then their arc swings

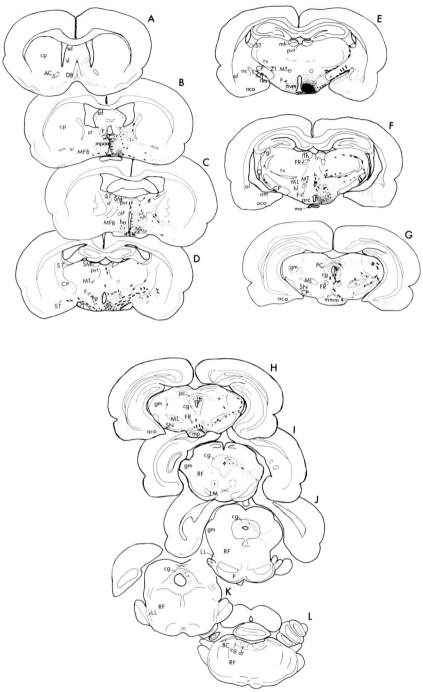

Figure 8–3. Distribution of labeled projections from an injection site in the ventromedial nucleus of the hypothalamus. Symbols as in Figure 8–1. (From Krieger et al., 1979)

medially again as they descend. These fibers cross the thalamic reticular nucleus at posterior levels. Some fibers continue to travel medially and terminate just lateral to the habenula. Others, more caudal, pass through and around the medial geniculate body and terminate near the central gray, including the area dorsal and lateral to the posterior commissure. In general, these laterally descending projections appear to be responsible for terminations in the mesencephalic reticular formation lateral to the central gray.

Other fibers descending from the ventromedial nucleus continue directly posteriorly through the hypothalamus, forming a "medial descending" fiber group. They run through premammillary and mammillary levels, joining the periventricular system as they travel dorsally toward the central gray. They form a strong projection to the central gray, especially to its dorsal and lateral portions. This projection continues as far posterior as the pontine central gray, medial to the locus ceruleus. This is the most posterior projection from the ventromedial nucleus of the hypothalamus that has been observed.

Ventromedial nucleus neurons also send projections to the median eminence (Krieger et al., 1979).

The lateral-going and medial-going groups of ventromedial nucleus fibers descending to the midbrain are the obvious candidates for fibers having the greatest role in the control of lordosis behavior. In subsequent studies, we analyzed the nature of their participation using transection methods (Chapter 9).

E. Arcuate Nucleus

Charts from tritiated amino acid autoradiograms showing the full pattern of axonal projections from the arcuate nucleus of the hypothalamus (Krieger et al., 1979) are presented in Figure 8–4.

Long axons projections from neurons in the arcuate nucleus are very light. They ascend primarily through the medial anterior hypothalamus and medial preoptic area in the periventricular system. Some axons reach the bed nucleus of the stria terminalis and as far anterior as the lateral septum. Very few axons go laterally into the supraoptic commissure. Similarly, the lateral projection through the zone incerta is very weak.

Some fibers descend medially through the posterior hypothalamus, with a few medial descending fibers entering the periventricular system and terminating in the lateral central gray. This is a very weak projection compared to that from the ventromedial nucleus.

Arcuate nucleus cells clearly project into the median eminence. Clumps of silver grains representing labeled fibers as well as scattered silver grains representing apparent fields of termination in the median eminence were obvious.

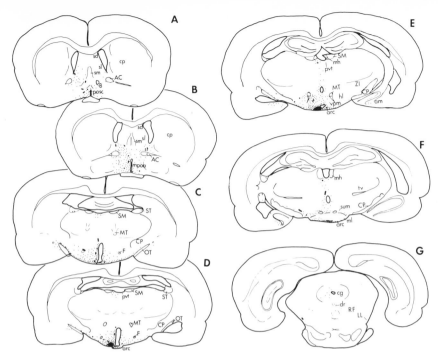

Figure 8–4. Distribution of labeled projections from an injection site in the arcuate nucleus of the hypothalamus. Symbols as in Figure 8–1. (From Krieger et al., 1979)

F.   Some Limbic Efferents

For comparison to hypothalamic efferents, especially with respect to paths taken by descending axons, we consider briefly projections from a few neighboring structures. Two points can be made: First, neighboring structures outside the hypothalamus and preoptic area proper have different patterns of projections from hypothalamic cell groups. Second, the paths taken by axons descending in and around the median forebrain bundle lend themselves to an orderly pattern of descending axons (Section G).

Neurons in the nuclei of the diagonal band of Broca have a grossly different pattern of projection from preoptic or hypothalamic neurons (Table 8-1). Axons from these neurons descending toward the midbrain run, in terms of medial–lateral position, in the middle of the medial forebrain bundle, outside of (i.e., lateral to) those from the medial preoptic area (Conrad and Pfaff, 1976a). In terms of dorsal–ventral position, they run at the bottom of the brain, below axons from the nucleus accumbens (Conrad and Pfaff, 1976a).

Axons descending from the nucleus accumbens run in the dorsal and lateral quadrant of the medial forebrain bundle (Conrad and Pfaff, 1976c).

At more caudal hypothalamic levels, nucleus accumbens axons in the medial forebrain bundle form a continuous distribution with labeled axons from the same structure that had been descending among fibers of the cerebral peduncle. Axons descending from neurons in the medial septum run in the medial forebrain bundle in a position similar to that taken by axons from the nuclei of the diagonal band of Broca (Conrad and Pfaff, 1976c). This makes sense. Septal axons pass through the diagonal bands of Broca on their way to the medial forebrain bundle. From our work it appears that the nucleus accumbens resembles the septum in its projections to some regions of the hypothalamus, thalamus, ventral tegmental area, and central gray, but is similar to the striatum in projecting to the globus pallidus, entopeduncular nucleus, and substantia nigra. Thus, although separate cases have been made on the basis of lesion evidence and developmental patterns for classification of nucleus accumbens with septum or striatum, from our neuroanatomical evidence it appears that the nucleus accumbens should be considered as intermediate between these two structures (Conrad and Pfaff, 1976c).

Projections from the olfactory tubercule have been studied extensively by Scott and his colleagues (Scott and Pfaffmann, 1967, 1972; Scott and Pfaff, 1970; Scott and Chafin, 1975). They found that axons from large neuronal cell bodies deep in the olfactory tubercule descend through the medial forebrain bundle in its ventral and lateral corner.

G.   Orderliness of Descending Axons: "Laminar Flow"

Principles of organization of fiber systems descending through the hypothalamus and medial forebrain bundle follow from the analyses of projections from preoptic, hypothalamic, and neighboring limbic structures (Pfaff and Conrad, 1978). First, more medially placed neurons have axons that tend to descend medially. Axons of more lateral neurons run more laterally. Second, the concept of an orderly medial–lateral arrangement (and dorsal–ventral arrangement) of fibers descending through and nearby the hypothalamus can be extended to an anterior–posterior concept ("laminar flow") by analyzing projections from regions bordering the preoptic area and hypothalamus.

1.   Medial–Lateral and Dorsal–Ventral Organization

The nucleus of the stria terminalis borders on the preoptic area dorsally. Its projections are, with a few exceptions, similar to those of the medial preoptic area (Conrad and Pfaff, 1976a). Axons descending from the bed nucleus of the stria terminalis run in the medial portion of the medial forebrain bundle. Importantly, however, they run in a position generally *dorsal* to that of medial preoptic axons; i.e., in contrast to preoptic axons, some bed nucleus of stria terminalis axons descending in the medial forebrain bundle run in a position dorsal to the fornix, and very few nucleus of stria terminalis axons course in the ventral hypothalamus. Furthermore, axons from the dorsomedial nucleus of the hypothalamus descend in a relatively dorsal position (Conrad and Pfaff, unpublished data)—hence the idea that axons from dorsally located neurons in and around the hypothalamus and preoptic area tend to descend in a relatively dorsal position.

We also found an orderly medial–lateral arrangement of descending axons in the hypothalamus and medial forebrain bundle. For neurons in both the medial preoptic area and the anterior hypothalamus, those cell bodies that are located most medially (in the periventricular strata) tend to have axons that ran more medially than those cell bodies located more laterally in the same cell groups (Conrad and Pfaff, 1976a,b). These comparisons are fully illustrated in the primary publications (Conrad and Pfaff, 1976a,b). For instance, the most medial and periventricular preoptic and anterior hypothalamic neuronal cell bodies give rise to axons that run in the periventricular zone of the hypothalamus, as well as to axons descending in the medial forebrain bundle or in the fiber bundle ventromedial to the fornix. Furthermore, the most medial and periventricular preoptic and anterior hypothalamic cell bodies run relatively heavier projections to the arcuate nucleus and the median eminence than do more laterally placed preoptic and anterior hypothalamic neurons. Extending this idea, the positions of axons descending from the paraventricular nucleus fit with the notion of an orderly medial–lateral arrangement of descending hypothalamic axons. Paraventricular axons, arising from their medially placed cell bodies, tend to remain medial, running in the periventricular zone of the hypothalamus and in the medial ventral hypothalamus. In this respect, they are similar to the axons of the most medial preoptic and anterior hypothalamic neurons. Thus, within the preoptic area and hypothalamus, more medially placed cell bodies have stronger medial (and weaker lateral) axonal trajectories in their descending projections.

Analyzing the pathway descending from neuronal cell bodies in the nucleus in the diagonal band of Broca, nucleus accumbens, and olfactory tubercule gives further support to the idea of orderliness in these descending projections as mentioned above (Conrad and Pfaff, 1976a,c). Axons from the diagonal band and nucleus accumbens neurons descend in the medial forebrain bundle. Diagonal band axons run in a very ventral position. Axons from nucleus accumbens, which start from more dorsally placed cell bodies, descend more dorsally in the medial forebrain bundle.

A schematic section through the hypothalamus is presented in Figure 8–5 to show the positions of these descending axons groups and their relation to each other. From this illustration it is clear that axons of

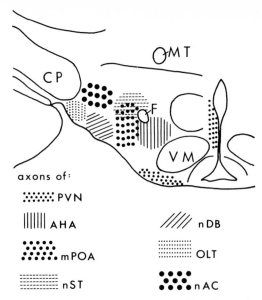

Figure 8–5. Relative positions of axons descending from the paraventricular nucleus *(PVN)*, anterior hypothalamic area (*AHA*), medial preoptic area (*mPOA*), bed nucleus of the stria terminalis (*nST*), nuclei of the diagonal band of Broca (*nDB*), olfactory tubercle (*OLT*), nucleus accumbens (*nAC*), and neurons in the hypothalamus and medial forebrain bundle at the level of the ventromedial nucleus. *CP,* cerebral peduncle; *F,* fornix; *MT,* mammillothalamic tract; *VM,* ventromedial nucleus. (From Pfaff & Conrad, 1978)

more medially located neuron cell bodies (for instance, the paraventricular nucleus, periventricular preoptic area, and periventricular anterior hypothalamus) run medially. Those of relatively dorsally located neuron cell bodies run more dorsally (for instance, the bed nucleus of stria terminalis and nucleus accumbens). Those from more ventrally located neurons run ventrally (for instance, the nuclei of the diagonal band and the olfactory tubercule). In conclusion, axons descending through the hypothalamus and medial forebrain bundle tend to be ordered among medial–lateral and dorsal–ventral gradients.

2. Anterior–Posterior Organization: Laminar Flow

Extending this idea of orderly descending axon trajectories to include anterior–posterior comparisons, it appears that efferents descending from the hypothalamus, preoptic area, and basal forebrain run in a spatial arrangement that resembles laminar flow (Figure 8–6); that is, the relative anterior–posterior level of the neuron cell bodies of origin (as well as their dorsal–ventral and medial–lateral position) determines the position their axons take in descending through the hypothalamus and medial

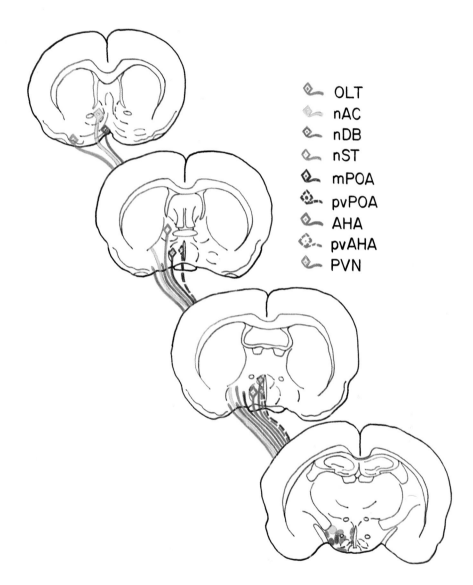

Figure 8–6. Laminar flow of axons descending from the paraventricular nucleus (*PVN*), anterior hypothalamus (*AHA*), medial preoptic area (*mPOA*), bed nucleus of the stria terminalis (*nST*), nuclei of the diagonal band (*nDB*), nucleus accumbens (*nAC*), and olfactory tubercle (*OLT*) through the medial basal forebrain, hypothalamus, and medial forebrain bundle. (From Pfaff & Conrad, 1978)

forebrain bundle (Pfaff and Conrad, 1978). The more anterior the cells of origin, the further lateral the axons tend to run (Figure 8–6). For instance, starting from the lateral side, axons from nerve cell bodies in the olfactory tubercule run in the ventrolateral corner of the medial forebrain bundle. Similarly, axons from cells in the nucleus accumbens run quite laterally. Axons from cell bodies that are placed more posteriorly, i.e., in the nucleus of the diagonal band of Broca, course medial to those from the olfactory tubercule. Further in, axons from the medial preoptic area and bed nucleus of stria terminalis nurons (located roughly at the same anterior–posterior level as each other) course in the most medial part of the medial forebrain bundle. Further posterior, axons from nerve cell bodies of the anterior hypothalamus run medial to those preoptic axons, not in the medial forebrain bundle proper but in a bundle ventral and medial to the fornix. Finally, paraventricular nucleus axons, arising from neurons posterior to the preoptic area, run even farther medially in the hypothalamus. Looking at the same organization from medial to lateral, we can say that axonal sheets from more anteriorly placed neurons are "wrapped around" (successively laterally) the descending axons sheets from more posteriorly placed structures.

Axons from the ventromedial nucleus of the hypothalamus travel in two groups. The lateral-going group of descending axons cuts across the medial forebrain bundle and also cuts across the principles of organization described above (Krieger et al., 1979). However, the medial-going group of descending axons from the ventromedial nucleus starts from a relatively posterior position in the preoptic–hypothalamic continuum and heads straight back through the hypothalamus, medial to any of the groups described above (Krieger et al., 1979). Thus, these axons conform to the laminar flow concept that more posteriorly placed nerve cell bodies give rise to axons descending in a more medial position.

We emphasize that this organization has been derived for axons descending from cell groups in the basal forebrain, preoptic area, and hypothalamus back through the level of the ventromedial nucleus. The descending axon groups are not completely discrete, as in a classically lemniscal system; rather, there is some overlap among the positions of descending axons from the brain regions discussed. The principles of organization of axons descending through the hypothalamus and medial forebrain bundle are derived from the relatively predominant positions of these axons.

3.   Conclusions

On the basis of the data reviewed above, we conclude that two organizing principles are at work on axons descending through the hypothalamus and medial forebrain bundle. The first is a tendency toward simple medial–lateral and dorsal–ventral organization. Axons from more medial neurons descend medially, and axons from ventral neurons run more ventrally. The second is a more complex tendency toward anterior–posterior organization, in which axons of more anterior neurons are wrapped laterally around the axon groups from more posterior neurons. Taken together, these tendencies result in a layering of fibers as they descend through the medial forebrain bundle and hypothalamus, in the manner of laminar flow (Figure 8–6). Axons from more anterior neurons in basal forebrain structures enter the medial forebrain bundle as far laterally as possible. Axons of progressively more posterior neurons "are laid into" the medial forebrain bundle, taking positions as far lateral as permitted by the descending fibers already there. Axons descending from neurons still further posterior, continue to "lay in" on the medial edge of axons aleady present. However, these axons do not run in the medial forebrain bundle itself, but through the medial hypothalamus (Pfaff and Conrad, 1978). These descriptions fit nicely with medial–lateral gradients in hypothalamic cell division leading to the final placement of hypothalamic cell bodies during development (Altman and Bayer, 1978a,b; Bayer and Altman, 1978).

Orderly arrangements of axons descending from the hypothalamus, preoptic area, and basal forebrain, as pointed out above, should help us in forming theories of hypothalamic development and hypothalamic organization, and should also help us to put functional investigations on a more sound anatomical footing. In particular, they lend perspective to the neuroanatomical circuitry proven to be of relevance for the control of reproductive behavior.

H. Summary

Using the tritiated amino acid autoradiographic technique, we have discovered long-ranging projections from medial preoptic and medial hypothalamic neurons. These are longer axoned trajectories than would have been suspected from the results of previous methodologies. They are not consistent with the idea that hypothalamic neurons are limited to control of the pituitary. Instead, projections to other brain regions can be found and presumably are involved in the control of behavior. Therefore, we can say that hypothalamic outflow serves to coordinate behavioral events and endocrine events, or vice versa.

Principles of organization of axons descending from the preoptic area and hypothalamus can be discerned. Within the hypothalamus, preoptic area, and basal forebrain, axons exiting from more medially placed cell bodies tend to have stronger medial trajectories. Axons exiting from more dorsally placed cell bodies tend to have stronger dorsal trajectories.

Sheets of axons from more anteriorly placed cell bodies tend to be wrapped more laterally as they descend through and around the medial forebrain bundle in the manner of a laminar flow.

The axons from the ventromedial nucleus of the hypothalamus descending to the midbrain are likely to be the most important for the control of lordosis behavior. These form two groups, one circling far laterally and then descending to the midbrain, the other going straight back through the medial hypothalamus and joining the periventricular system.

Chapter 9

Midbrain Module

Since decerebrate female rats with complete transections between dien-cephalon and mesencephalon do not perform lordosis (Figure 7–11; Kow et al., 1978), an output descending from the diencephalon or telence-phalon must be required for mediating the behavior. Anterior to these complete transections, no source of axons other than the ventromedial nucleus of the hypothalamus has been shown to be necessary for lordosis (Chapter 7). Moreover, a common route of output from the diencephalon and mesencephalon, the medial forebrain bundle, does not carry descend-ing ventromedial nucleus axons and is not required for lordosis (Modianos et al., 1976). Thus it appears that only output descending from neurons in and around the ventromedial nucleus of the hypothalamus is necessary for the behavior to occur. Presumably, these axons carry the estrogenic influences that mark control by the hormone over the behavior.

By far the largest number of axons from the ventromedial nucleus end in or near the central gray of the mesencephalon. Thus nerve cells in and near the central gray are the best candidates for relaying descending hypothalamic control. We analyzed which axons from the ventromedial nucleus to central gray might be important for lordosis behavior by transecting them selectively (Section A). In turn, limitations on the length of axons involved allow us to prove the existence of a midbrain module in the control of lordosis behavior (Section B). Similarly, anatomical limitations on the length of axons descending from the midbrain allow us to prove the existence of a medullary module in lordosis control. In the midbrain itself, we used electrical stimulation and lesion techniques to study the participation of central gray cells (Section C). Then we could describe some of the properties of relevant cells in the central gray using extracellular single unit recording (Section D). Finally, we have de-scribed, in anatomical terms, the output descending from midbrain central gray neurons as far as the medulla, forming the input to a medullary module in lordosis control (Section E).

A.   From Hypothalamus to Midbrain

Fibers from the ventromedial nucleus of the hypothalamus enter the midbrain over either of two well-defined trajectories, one medial (periventricular), the other sweeping laterally (Figure 8–3; Conrad and Pfaff, 1976b; Krieger et al., 1979). We studied the contributions to lordosis by fibers descending through these two trajectories by transecting them selectively (Manogue et al., 1980a). When the lateral-running fibers are intact, the medial-running fibers are not necessary for lordosis to occur (Figure 9–1). Although not necessary, the medial fibers do contribute to lordosis control because they can substitute for the lateral fibers (see below), and under some conditions medial fiber lesions lead to temporary lordosis deficits (Sakuma, Edwards, and Pfaff, 1980). When the medial-running fibers from the ventromedial nucleus are intact, the lateral-running fibers are not absolutely necessary for lordosis to occur (Manogue et al., 1980a). The results from a series of transections (in different rats) of the lateral fiber system, each nearly complete, clearly show that no single subset of these lateral fibers is essential for lordosis behavior. Nevertheless, fibers running laterally from the ventromedial nucleus certainly contribute to lordosis behavior, since their destruction can lead to large deficits. Lordosis losses appear whether the lateral fibers are transected with a sagittal knife cut, near the ventromedial nucleus (Figure 9–2), or, farther posterior, with knife cuts in a transverse plane (Figure 9–3). Because the quantitative losses are larger following lateral than medial transections, the former appear to play a quantitatively greater role in lordosis behavior control. Whether the reason is that larger numbers of ventromedial nucleus axons travel the lateral route, or that they play a more crucial functional role independent of axon number, we do not yet know.

Thus, lordosis behavior control by axons from the ventromedial nucleus of the hypothalamus to the midbrain central gray take the form of an asymmetrical (OR) gate. Both medial- and lateral-running fibers participate, and to some extent they can substitute for each other. Quantitatively, however, the lateral-running fibers appear to play a larger part.

B.   Proof of Modules in Brainstem

We can deduce something of the nature of brainstem modules for controlling lordosis from anatomical limitations on axon length. Briefly, since ventromedial neuronal axons do not project past midbrain, there must be a midbrain module; and, since midbrain neurons in the target regions of hypothalamic axons (i.e., in and around the central gray) do not send axons to the spinal cord and do to the medulla, there must be a medullary module.

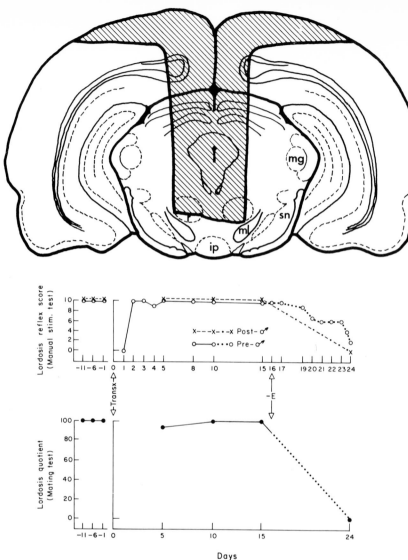

Figure 9–1. Transection of only the medial-running axons from the ventromedial hypothalamus to the midbrain central gray did not disrupt lordosis. *E:* removal of estrogen. (From Manogue et al., 1980a)

First, to prove the existence of a midbrain module we know from tritiated amino acid autoradiography that axons descending from neurons in and around the ventromedial nucleus of the hypothalamus do not extend beyond the mesencephalon (Conrad and Pfaff, 1976b; Krieger et al., 1979). Therefore, there must be a module of mesencephalic neurons, the midbrain module, that is importantly involved in the control of lordosis by carrying hormone-dependent hypothalamic influences.

Within the midbrain, the anatomical distribution of terminals of

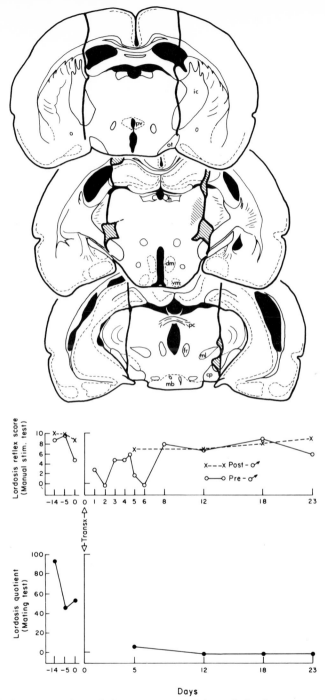

Figure 9–2. Transection of the ventromedial hypothalamic axons running laterally in a trajectory which ends in and near the central gray reduced lordosis (especially in response to a male) but did not abolish it. (From Manogue et al., 1980a)

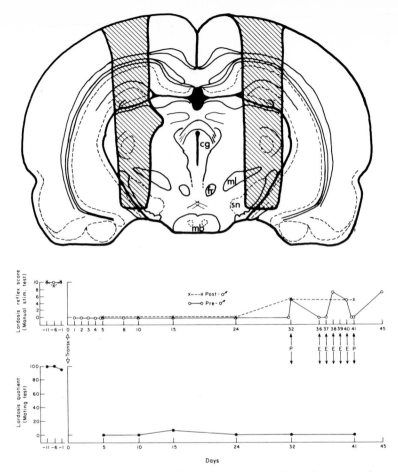

Figure 9–3. Deep bilateral transections that cut lateral-running axons from the ventromedial hypothalamus severely reduced lordosis performance, although the reflex could still be performed. *E*, supplementary estrogen; *P*, tests following progesterone. (From Manogue et al., 1980a)

hypothalamic axons indicates the locations of those brainstem nerve cell bodies that are candidates for relaying or transforming hypothalamic lordosis-controlling signals. Mesencephalic neurons receiving axonal projections from the ventromedial hypothalamic nucleus (and from anterior hypothalamus) are in the central gray, the dorsal mesencephalic reticular formation and cuneiform nucleus adjacent to the central gray, and the magnocellular division of the medial geniculate body (Conrad and Pfaff, 1976b; Krieger et al., 1979).

Second, to prove the existence of a module in the medulla we have autoradiographic and HRP evidence. Tritiated amino acid autoradiography applied to studying the descending projections from the very mesencephalic regions mentioned above, in and near the central gray, shows that axons from these neurons do not reach the spinal cord (Krieger and

Pfaff, 1980; Ruda, 1976). In a complementary study, HRP was applied to severed axons in columns in the spinal cord, following HRP treatment of axons at low thoracic levels. No retrograde-filled cells were found in or around the midbrain central gray (Zemlan et al., 1978). This result also shows that these midbrain cells do not project to the spinal cord. Therefore, there must be a block of neurons in the lower brainstem that carry mesencephalic lordosis-relevant, hormone-dependent influences (which, in turn, had originated in the hypothalamus).

The mesencephalic neurons involved do send descending axons that terminate in the nucleus gigantocellularis in the medullary reticular formation. Anatomical work with both the mesencephalic central gray (Hamilton and Skultety, 1970; Ruda, 1976) and rats (Krieger and Pfaff, 1980) and the mesencephalic cuneiform nucleus (Edwards, 1975; Edwards and de Olmos, 1976) has shown projections descending to the region of medullary reticulospinal neurons. In fact, cells in the midbrain central gray of the rat can be antidromically stimulated from the reticular formation of the medulla (Sakuma and Pfaff, 1980c). In turn, as shown by lesion studies, these reticulospinal neurons are important in the performance of lordosis (Modianos and Pfaff, 1976b, 1979).

Thus, there must be at least a mesencephalic block and a medullary block of neurons involved in descending lordosis control. Relevant hypothalamic neurons synapse on the mesencephalic neurons designated above. These neurons, in turn, synapse in the ventral portion of the nucleus gigantocellularis of the medulla. Reticulospinal neurons in this region can then influence lordosis mechanisms in the spinal cord.

Since rats with complete spinal transections do not perform lordosis (Pfaff et al., 1972; Kow et al., 1977; Kow et al., 1980b), the net influence of descending axons from the medulla on the spinal cord must be facilitatory for lordosis. As mentioned above, the net influence of hypothalamic output to the midbrain is also facilitatory for lordosis. Taken together, these two demonstrations place limitations on the signs of synaptic effects in the brainstem. We know (see above) that there must be at least two levels of synapses, one in the mesencephalon and the other in the medulla. These must preserve, from the hypothalamus to the spinal cord, the relationship that increased activity leads to increased lordosis. Therefore, if the net synaptic effect in the mesencephalon is excitatory, that in the medulla also must be excitatory. Likewise, if the net synaptic effect in the mesencepahlon is inhibitory, that in the medulla also must be inhibitory.

If sources of lordosis-relevant fibers from the diencephalon must be in and around the ventromedial nucleus, then only axons from those sources could be important. Therefore, the limitations on the terminal fields of those axons descending to the midbrain, namely in and around the central gray of the midbrain, show that only those locations in the midbrain could be primarily important for lordosis. This deduction is strongly supported by the lesion and stimulation evidence presented in

Section D. In turn, the retrograde neuroanatomical technique of HRP applications in and around the midbrain central gray would be expected to show cell bodies in and around the ventromedial hypothalamic nucleus, which include those governing lordosis. Indeed, following central gray HRP applications, cells in the ventromedial hypothalamic nucleus are filled (Morrell, Greenberger, and Pfaff, 1978, 1980). However, when this type of HRP experiment is combined with estrogen autoradiography, no double-labeled cells are seen (Chapter 6); that is, there is not yet clear evidence that those cells which concentrate estrogen project from the ventromedial nucleus to the central gray. Therefore, it seems likely that estrogen-concentrating cells in and around the ventromedial nucleus of the hypothalamus have their primary action on lordosis by local projections (Figure 6–10).

In summary, at least two brainstem modules relay hormone-dependent, lordosis-controlling signals from the ventromedial hypothalamus to the spinal cord. One set of such neurons comprises a midbrain module in an around the mesencephalic central gray. The other set of neurons comprises a medullary module located at least in the ventral portion of the nucleus gigantocellularis in the medullary reticular formation.

C.   Midbrain Central Gray Stimulation Enhances Lordosis; Lesions Disrupt It

Electrical stimulation in and adjacent to the midbrain central gray in anesthetized female rats can yield tail, tailbase, and rump movements that use the same muscle groups as lordosis behavior (Figure 9–4; Pfaff et al., 1972). These results led to the hypothesis that midbrain central gray neurons are involved in facilitating lordosis behavior; this hypothesis has been confirmed by several lines of experimental evidence.

Electrical stimulation of the central gray facilitates lordosis behavior in normal, freely moving female rats (Sakuma and Pfaff, 1979a). In contrast to ventromedial hypothalamic stimulation, the behavioral effect of midbrain central gray stimulation is immediate (Figure 9–5). Considerably higher frequencies are effective, compared to those for hypothalamic stimulation (Figure 9–6). Currents as low as 10 μA were adequate. Nevertheless, it is striking that electrical stimulation of the central gray does not substitute for estrogen in promoting lordosis behavior (Figure 9–7).

Ventromedial hypothalamic projections to the central gray show the anatomical substrate for central gray control of lordosis. Electrical stimulation has shown that neurons there are sufficient to facilitate this behavior. Lesion results suggest that in some aspects these neurons are essential. Electrolytic bilateral lesions in the central gray result in a decrement in lordosis scores (Sakuma and Pfaff, 1979b). In contrast to

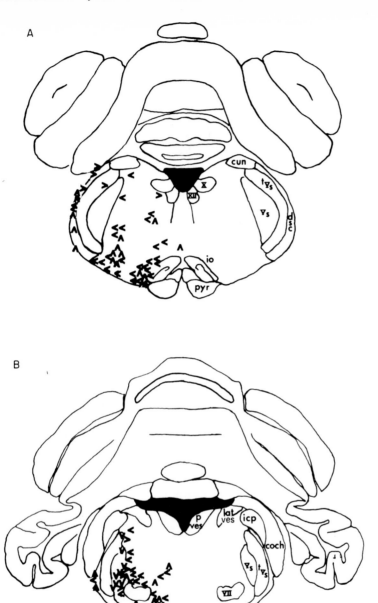

Figure 9–4. Points in female rat brain from which tail, tailbase, or rump movements can be electrically stimulated under anesthesia. <, movement to ipsilateral; >, movement to contralateral; ∧ , elevation. (From Pfaff et al., 1972) *Abbreviations: ac,* anterior commissure; *aco,* cortical amygdaloid nucleus; *am,* medial amygdaloid nucleus; *bic,* brachium of the inferior colliculus; *caud,* caudate-putamen; *cc,* corpus callosum; *cg,* central gray; *coch,* ventral cochlear nucleus; *cun,* cuneate nucleus; *dg,* dentate gyrus of the hippocampus; *dsc,* dorsal

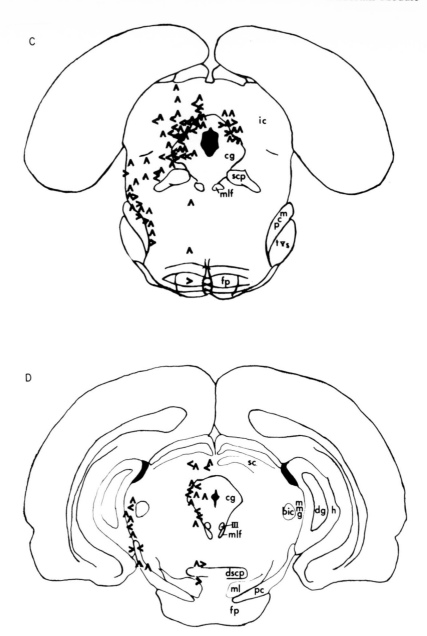

spinocerebellar tract; *dscp*, decussation of the superior cerebellar peduncle; *f*,
fornix; *fp*, frontopontine fibers; *h*, hippocampus (Ammon's horn); *hi*, habenulointerpeduncular tract; *ic*, inferior colliculus; *icp*, inferior cerebellar peduncle;
io, inferior olive; *lat ves*, lateral vestibular nucleus; *lot*, lateral olfactory tract; *m*,
mammillary bodies; *mcp*, middle cerebellar peduncle; *mfb*, medial forebrain
bundle; *ml*, medial lemniscus; *mlf*, medial longitudinal fasciculus; *mmg*, magnocellular medial geniculate body; *mpoa*, medial preoptic area; *mt*, mammillothal-

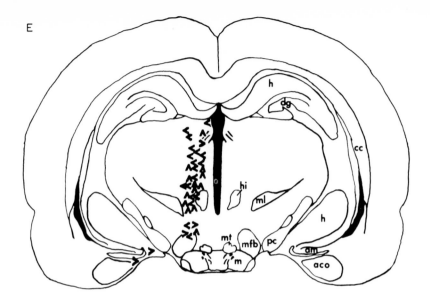

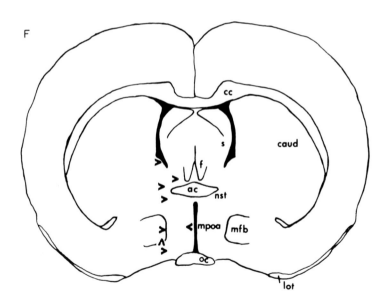

amic tract; *nst*, nucleus of the stria terminalis; *oc*, optic chiasm; *pc*, cerebral
peduncle; *p ves*, principal vestibular nucleus; *pyr*, pyramidal tract; *s*, septum; *sc*,
superior colliculus; *scp*, superior cerebellar peduncle; *III*, nucleus of the oculomotor nerve; *Vs*, nucleus of spinal radiation of the trigeminal nerve; *tVs*, spinal
radiation of the trigeminal nerve; *VII*, nucleus of the facial nerve; *X*, dorsal
motor nucleus of the vagus nerve; *XII*, nucleus of the hypoglossal nerve.

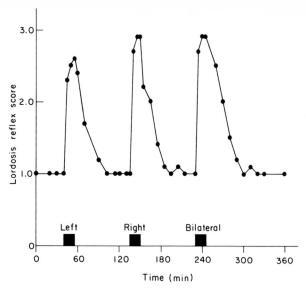

Figure 9–5. Electrical stimulation of the central gray facilitated lordosis behavior. (From Sakuma & Pfaff, 1979a)

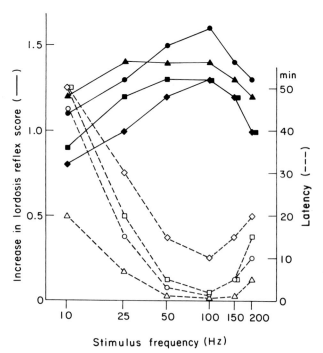

Figure 9–6. Optimum frequencies for lordosis facilitation from the central gray were between 50 and 150 Hz. (From Sakuma & Pfaff, 1979a)

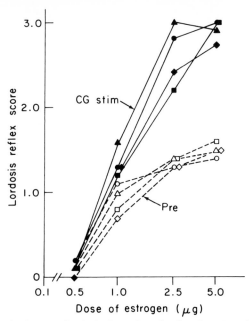

Figure 9–7. Lordosis magnitude before (*Pre, broken lines*) and during (*CG stim, solid lines*) stimulation of central gray as a function of estrogen dose. (From Sakuma & Pfaff, 1979a)

ventromedial hypothalamic lesions, the behavior decrement following central gray destruction is immediate (Figure 9–8). Lesions that destroy the dorsal central gray lead to the most severe losses of lordosis. Ventromedial hypothalamic lesions still allow electrical stimulation of the central gray to lead to lordosis enhancement; however, central gray lesions abolish the ability of ventromedial hypothalamic stimulation to facilitate lordosis behavior (Sakuma and Pfaff, 1979b). Thus, the ventromedial hypothalamic influence probably does act, as hypothesized, through central gray neurons.

Destruction of midbrain tissue just outside the central gray, on the border between the central gray and the cuneiform nucleus, reduces both lordosis behavior itself and the ability of central gray stimulation to enhance it (Figure 9–9). We presume that important central gray axons exit through this region, traveling posteriorly.

In contrast, lesions more lateral in the dorsal midbrain can lead to lordosis losses without harming the ability of central gray stimulation to enhance the behavior (Sakuma and Pfaff, 1979b). Carrer (1978) also found that more laterally placed lesions, just medial to the medial geniculate body, can lead to lordosis decrements. Midbrain tissue destruction with his technique probably is similar to the deep laterally placed transections that Manogue et al. (1980a) found lead to severe lordosis losses (Figure 9–3). Such destruction not only cuts lordosis-relevant somatosensory input to the midbrain (Zemlan, et al 1978), but

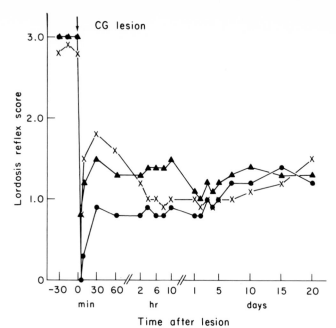

Figure 9–8. Time course of lordosis loss following lesion of central gray (*CG*) in each of three female rats. (From Sakuma & Pfaff, 1979b)

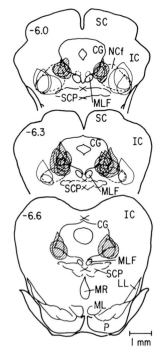

Figure 9–9. Bilateral lesions (*hatched areas*) on the ventrolateral borders of central gray (*CG*) not only reduced lordosis but also the behavior-facilitating effect of central gray stimulation. (From Sakuma & Pfaff, 1979b)

also destroys, at least in part, lateral-running fibers descending from the ventromedial hypothalamus (Krieger et al., 1979). When placed posteriorly enough, these laterally located lesions or transections might even sever axons descending from the central gray (Ruda, 1976).

D. Electrophysiological Properties of Midbrain Cells Relevant to Lordosis Control and Estrogen Effects

Nerve cells receive inputs, transform those inputs in some way, and produce an output. Under this formulation, two actions that midbrain cells could do relevant to lordosis control would be to transform estrogen-dependent ventromedial hypothalamic signals in such a way as to form an output to the lower brainstem and to transform ascending lordosis-relevant somatosensory information by way of participating in an upper reflex loop. The ventromedial hypothalamic hormone-dependent information coming to the midbrain is essential for lordosis. There are cells in the central gray whose electrophysiological properties seem to show that they specialize in receiving and transforming such information. They are described below in Section 1. Somatosensory input to midbrain neurons is probably less important for reflex control on a lordosis-by-lordosis basis. Some reasons for this were mentioned in Chapter 5, Section D.2. Nevertheless, some cells do respond to interesting somatosensory stimuli, as described below in Section 2.

1. Electrophysiology of Midbrain Cells Projecting to the Medulla: Hormonal and Hypothalamic Effects on Them

Nerve cells in the midbrain central gray have been antidromically identified by electrical stimulation in nucleus gigantocellularis in the reticular formation of the medulla (Sakuma and Pfaff, 1980b). Conventional criteria for antidromic identification, including collision, were used (Figure 9–10). Large numbers of neuronal cell bodies thus identified were located in the midbrain central gray (Figure 9–11). These cells did not respond strongly or promptly to somatosensory stimulation, including stimuli that are relevant for the control of lordosis behavior.

Ventromedial hypothalamic stimulation and estrogen had significant electrophysiological effects on these cells. Two types of units were found and contrasted with each other, based on spike duration. As opposed to fast spikes, slow spikes had a very long spike duration. Especially in these slow units, it was possible to see and quantify the failures of antidromically stimulated spikes to propogate in the soma (Sakuma and

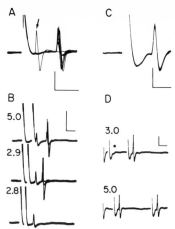

Figure 9–10 A–D. Antidromic identification of nerve cell bodies in midbrain central gray from electrical stimulation of their axons in medullary reticular formation. (A) Several antidromic spikes in a central gray cell. In one case a spontaneous orthodromic action potential (*arrow*) proved the antidromic nature of the medullary stimulated spikes, through collision. (B) Facilitation of central gray spike by second medullary stimulus, and dependence of this on interstimulus interval. (C) Antidromic spike in another cell, with a "fast" spike (no notch, short duration, short antidromic latency). (D) At 3.0–millisecond interval following spontaneous spike, antidromic spike was blocked by collision (dot). At 5.0–millisecond interval, it was not. (From Sakuma & Pfaff, 1980a)

Pfaff, 1980b). In fact, this quantification can be used as a measure of the electrical excitability of the cell body. Electrical stimulation of the ventromedial nucleus of the hypothalamus increased the excitability of midbrain central gray cell bodies thus measured (Figure 9–12; Sakuma and Pfaff, 1980b). Preoptic influences lowered the excitability of these midbrain central gray neurons. Estrogen increased the invasion of the

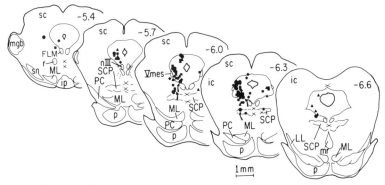

Figure 9–11. Locations of units in midbrain central gray that were antidromically identified from medullary reticular formation. (From Sakuma & Pfaff, 1980c)

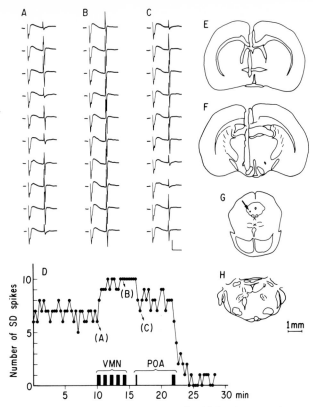

Figure 9–12 A –C. Antidromic stimulation of a midbrain central gray cell (location shown in G) from electrode in medullary reticular formation (location shown in H), with or without invasion of the soma and dendrites (*SD*), at times in the recording graphed in D. Electrical stimulation of the ventromedial hypothalamus (*VMN*, location shown in F) increased the central gray neuron's excitability, as measured by increased antidromic SD invasion. Preoptic stimulation (*POA*, location shown in E) decreased it. (From Sakuma & Pfaff, 1980b)

soma by antidromically stimulated spikes (i.e., increased cell body electrical excitability) and increased the resting discharge rate of some cells within the population of neurons in the midbrain central gray (Figure 9–13; Sakuma and Pfaff, 1980c).

Thus, influences that increase lordosis performance (ventromedial nucleus action and estrogen) increase the electrical excitability of these lordosis-facilitating midbrain central gray cells, and an influence that decreases lordosis (preoptic action) decreases the excitability of these cells. In turn, these cells facilitate lordosis (Section C. above). That fits. It is consistent with all of the above facts to say that estrogen promotes lordosis by increasing the activity of ventromedial hypothalamic cells and decreasing the activity of medial preoptic cells (Bueno and Pfaff, 1976). These hormone-induced alterations are then registered through the descending projections of these ventromedial hypothalamic and

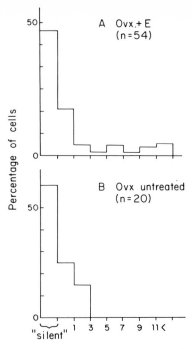

Figure 9–13. In estrogen-treated females (A) some midbrain central gray neurons had higher resting discharge rates than were ever seen in control untreated ovariectomized animals (B). (From Sakuma & Pfaff, 1980b)

medial preoptic cells to the central gray of the midbrain. Increased input there from the ventromedial hypothalamus and decreased input from the medial preoptic area would both act to increase the electrical excitability of midbrain central gray cells, which, in turn, promote lordosis behavior.

2. Responses to Somatosensory Input

The neuroanatomical basis for somatosensory input to the central gray and dorsal reticular formation of the midbrain has been described in Chapter 5 (Figure 5–4; Mehler, 1969; Zemlan et al., 1978). Indeed, neurons in and around the midbrain central gray can respond to somatosensory input which appears to be relevant to lordosis (Table 5–2; Malsbury et al., 1972; Pfaff, 1973). Subsequently, Carrer (1978) found evoked potentials in the laterally placed anterolateral column projection region (Zemlan et al., 1979) of the rat midbrain following electrical stimulation of the pudendal nerve. Latencies were often between 20 and 25 milliseconds. Among central gray cells that were *not* shown by antidromic stimulation to project to the medulla, we found more examples of midbrain cells responding to somatosensory input (Sakuma and Pfaff, 1980d). Cells with receptive fields confined to the perineal region were often found in the lateral and ventrolateral midbrain central gray. Cells with larger receptive fields either on the back or on both the dorsal and ventral surfaces of the body were often found in the dorsal and dorsolateral central gray.

Somatosensory input to midbrain central gray cells probably does not play the dominant role in the mechanism by which they control each lordosis response. First, no aspect of information ascending through the medial lemniscus system has been shown to be essential for lordosis. The dorsal columns (Kow et al., 1977), medial lemniscus, ventrolateral thalamus (Manogue et al., 1980a) and somatosensory cortex (Beach, 1944) all can be damaged or destroyed without lordosis loss. Cutaneous information ascending from the anterolateral columns to the midbrain may not be essential either. Transection of these columns as they enter the midbrain does not result in the lordosis losses that follow more anterior mesencephalic transections (Figure 9–14; Manogue et al., 1980a). Furthermore, those neurons most likely to be directly important for lordosis control—the cells that can be antidromically identified from the medullary reticular formation—do not show convincing responses to somatosensory stimulation (Sakuma and Pfaff, 1980b). Finally, in recent single unit recording experiments (Sakuma and Pfaff, 1980d), as before (Malsbury et al., 1972), estrogen had no effect on the responses of midbrain central gray cells to cutaneous input. Thus, rather than directing reproductive behavior control on a lordosis-by-lordosis basis through those midbrain neurons which are most powerfully and directly concerned, somatosensory input to the midbrain may play a more indirect role having to do with arousal states, leading to facilitation of reproductive behavior through multisynaptic descending routes.

3.   Synthesis

Midbrain nerve cells most likely to be powerfully and directly concerned with lordosis control are those in and near the central gray which can be antidromically stimulated from the medullary reticular formation. Hypothalamic influences and estrogen dominate the electrical excitability of those cells. This may occur through conventional synaptic mechanisms or through neuromodulatory actions of hypothalamically produced substances such as LHRH (see Chapter 7). Somatosensory input to these midbrain cells appears to have a less powerful and direct role.

E.   Output Descending from the Midbrain

At mesencephalic levels, descending fibers travel through or immediately adjacent to the central gray without actually forming a bundle (Hamilton and Skultety, 1970). At the posterior end of the mesencephalon, descend-

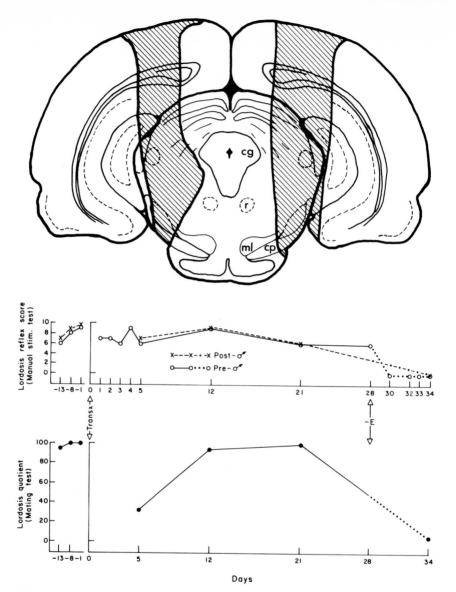

Figure 9–14. Deep lateral transections at posterior midbrain levels, cutting ascending anterolateral column fibers but not ventromedial hypothalamic fibers, did not abolish lordosis. −*E:* withdrawal of estrogen treatment. (From Manogue et al., 1980a)

ing fibers exit the central gray by turning laterally at its ventrolateral corner and heading out beneath the inferior colliculus, through the cuneiform nucleus (Hamilton and Skultety, 1970). As they head ventrolaterally and posteriorly, they are joined by fibers that exited the dorsal central gray at more anterior levels and descended at the posterior edge of the posterior commissure system (Ruda, 1976). These fibers project to the reticular formation of the lower brainstem. Their longest descending projection is most interesting. It leads to the reticular formation of the medulla, in the most ventral part of the nucleus gigantocellularis (Hamilton and Skultety, 1970; Ruda, 1976). In cats, a central gray projection extends to exactly that portion of the medullary reticular formation that contains reticulospinal cells projecting to lumbar levels (Zemlan et al., 1979); lesion of these cells leads to lordosis losses (Zemlan et al., 1980).

In rats, axons descending from the midbrain central gray have been demonstrated by tritiated amino acid autoradiography (Figure 9–15; Krieger and Pfaff, 1980). Some fibers reach the ventral portion of the nucleus gigantocellularis in the medullary reticular formation, mentioned above. This is the portion where reticulospinal cells projecting to the lumbar cord of the rat can be found (Zemlan et al., 1979). Connections from midbrain central gray, to medullary reticulospinal cells, to lumbar cord represent the shortest and simplest way by which midbrain cells could control lordosis behavior.

Projections from the central gray to the medullary reticular formation in the rat were also demonstrated electrophysiologically (see Section E; Sakuma and Pfaff, 1980b). Neurons with cell bodies in the midbrain central gray itself can be antidromically stimulated from the nucleus gigantocellularis (Figure 9–10).

The exact manner in which midbrain central gray cells participate in the control of lordosis remains to be discovered. It may be simpler than expected. For instance, Mori, Nishimura, Kurakami, et al. (1978) have suggested that midbrain activation of a spinal stepping generator in cats is a function of a simple increase of postural tonus.

No studies have shown any projections from the midbrain central gray to the lumbar spinal cord. There must be cell bodies in the lower brainstem (probably the ventral portion of the medullary reticular formation) that carry behaviorally relevant information to the cord.

The descending tracts which have been identified (Chapter 10) as controlling lordosis behavior are the lateral vestibulospinal tract (cell bodies in the lateral vestibular nucleus) and the lateral reticulospinal tract (cell bodies in the ventral medullary reticular formation). No studies have shown projections from the midbrain central gray to the lateral vestibular nucleus. Therefore, reticulospinal cells in the ventral medullary reticular formation are the most likely to carry the hormone-dependent hypothalamic output signals for controlling lordosis; these signals are first transformed and relayed in the midbrain central gray.

F.   Summary

Groups of cells in the midbrain central gray and medullary reticular formation form brainstem modules that control lordosis behavior. From the hypothalamus to the spinal cord they preserve the relationship that increased cellular activity leads to increased lordosis.

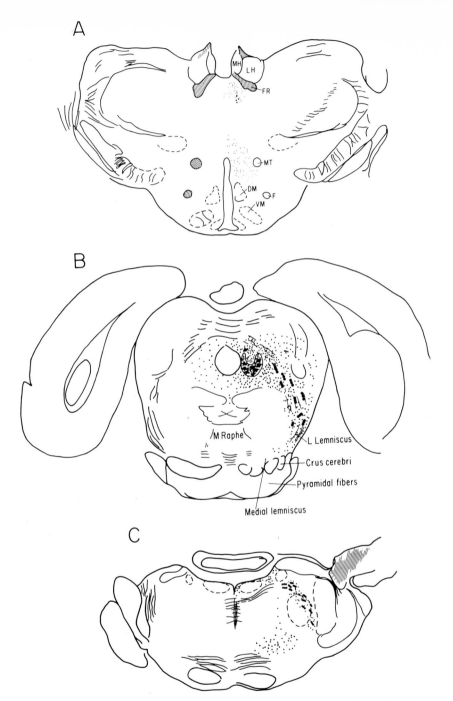

Figure 9–15 A–C. Some of the projections from midbrain central gray in the rat, as shown by tritiated amino acid autoradiography. (A) Labeled fibers (*dots*) ascending through the hypothalamus and thalamus. (B) Level with injection site. (C) Labeled fibers descending to and through the pontine reticular formation. Some reach the medulla. (From Krieger & Pfaff, 1980)

Axons from the ventromedial hypothalamus to the midbrain central gray travel either a medial or a lateral route. They comprise an asymmetrical OR gate with respect to lordosis control. To some extent, either can substitute for the other. However, the lateral-running fibers make the more important quantitative contribution (Figure 9–16).

Electrical stimulation in the midbrain central gray facilitates lordosis behavior. Central gray lesions disrupt it.

The electrical activity of many central gray neurons, including those that project to the medulla, is dominated by hypothalamic and hormonal influences. Estrogen and input from the ventromedial hypothalamic nucleus raise the excitability of these central gray nerve cells. Influences from the medial preoptic area lower it.

Somatosensory information of the sort related to lordosis behavior reaches midbrain neurons. However, it does not seem to have a direct or powerful role in the control of each lordosis response by midbrain central gray neurons. It may have a more general arousing function, indirectly related to lordosis behavior, which is transmitted to the lower brainstem over a multisynaptic route.

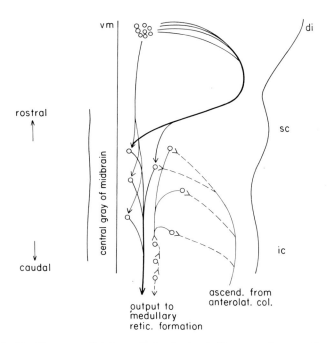

Figure 9–16. Ventromedial hypothalamic (*vm*) fibers project to the midbrain central gray by a medial and (more importantly for lordosis) a lateral trajectory. There, ventromedial influences increase the excitability of central gray neurons whose axons project to the medullary reticular formation. Cutaneous information, ascending from the anterolateral columns, does reach this midbrain region, but does not activate midbrain neurons whose axons reach the medulla. *di,* diencephalon; *sc,* level of superior colliculus; *ic,* level of inferior colliculus.

Midbrain central gray cells project to the reticular formation of the lower brainstem, including the ventral portion of the medullary reticular formation. Through contacts with reticulospinal cells in the ventral nucleus gigantocellularis, midbrain signals can be transferred to the spinal cord.

Part 3

Executive Control over the Behavior: Descending and Motor Pathways

Chapter 10

Brainstem to Spinal Cord

A. Descending Tracts to Be Considered

Female rats that have undergone complete transection of the spinal cord do not perform lordosis (Kow et al., 1977, 1980b). Therefore, control from the brainstem is obligatory, and its net effect must be to facilitate the behavior. Such descending fibers must run in the anterolateral columns (broadly defined), since these are necessary and sufficient for lordosis (Kow et al., 1977). The critical fibers must reach lumbar levels, since the crucial hindquarter movements are controlled from there (Chapter 11). The eight tracts classically recognized as descending from brainstem to spinal cord include the corticospinal, rubrospinal, tecto-spinal, isthmospinal, medial vestibulospinal, and medial reticulospinal, but the cell bodies and descending fibers of the lateral vestibulospinal tract and lateral reticulospinal tract (Figures 10–1 and 10–2) are of special interest (Zemlan and Pfaff, 1979; Zemlan et al., 1979).

B. Involvement of Descending Tracts in Lordosis

1. Tracts Not Involved

We begin deducing which descending tracts are involved in lordosis control by a process of elimination. The *corticospinal tract* cannot be crucial for lordosis behavior because its transection at spinal cord levels has no effect on lordosis (Kow, Montgomery, and Pfaff, 1973, 1977) and because lesions (Beach, 1944) or spreading depression (Clemens et al., 1967) of the cortical cell bodies giving rise to the corticospinal tract do not reduce the performance of lordosis. Bilateral surgical transections of

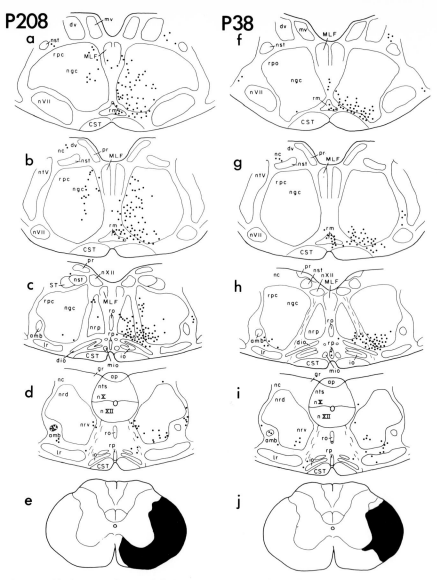

Figure 10–1. Locations of HRP-filled cell bodies (*dots*) in the rat medulla following transection and HRP application to lateral (*P38*) or ventral and lateral (*P208*) column fibers at cervical levels. (From Zemlan & Pfaff, 1979)

the entire dorsal half of the spinal cord at cervical or thoracic levels have no effect on lordosis; transections of the medial columns can be added to these and lordosis can still be performed (Kow et al., 1977). Besides eliminating the corticospinal tract from consideration, these transections also eliminate consideration of the *rubrospinal tract*. Since fibers of the rubrospinal tract run in the dorsal part of the lateral columns, they cannot be involved in any important way (Brown, 1974; Nyberg-Hansen, 1966;

Petras, 1967; Waldron and Gwyn, 1969). Similarly, *tectospinal fibers* can be eliminated from consideration because they run only in the medial columns and because they descend only to cervical levels (Nyberg-Hansen, 1966; Petras, 1967; Waldron and Gwyn, 1969). Likewise, the *interstitiospinal tract* is restricted to the medial columns (Nyberg-Hansen, 1966) and therefore can be transected without loss of lordosis.

The remaining tracts are the vestibulospinal and reticulospinal. The

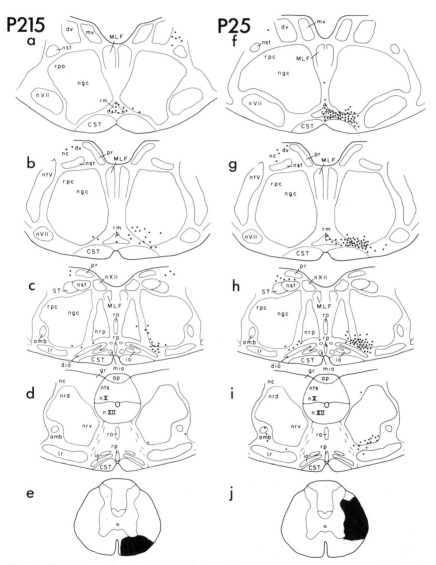

Figure 10–2. Locations of HRP-filled cell bodies in the rat medulla following transection and HRP application to lateral (*P25*) or ventral (*P215*) column fibers at low thoracic levels. Symbols as in Figure 10–1. (From Zemlan & Pfaff, 1979)

medial vestibulospinal tract runs in the medial columns and therefore is not primarily involved in lordosis (Nyberg-Hansen, 1964). Cell bodies giving rise to it can be lesioned without a change in lordosis behavior (Modianos and Pfaff, 1976b). The *medial reticulospinal tract* (from the pontine reticular formation) runs in the ventral columns (Nyberg-Hansen, 1965; Petras, 1967) and therefore can be eliminated from consideration.

We also know that the cerebellum does not play a major primary role in the control of lordosis-relevant pathways. Virtual removal of the cerebellum can be followed by strong lordosis reflexes in female rats (Zemlan and Pfaff, 1975). Destruction of the source of a major input to the cerebellum, the inferior olive, or major cerebellar output systems, the deep nuclei or the superior cerebellar peduncle, had no significant effect on lordosis in hormone-primed female rats (Modianos and Pfaff, 1976b).

2.   Tracts Involved

Following this process of elimination, the classical descending tracts remaining are the *lateral vestibulospinal tract* and the *lateral reticulospinal tract*. These are strong candidates for carrying the descending control of lordosis. The lateral vestibulospinal tract arises in the lateral vestibular nucleus (Deiter's nucleus) and its fibers run in the most ventral and medial part of the anterolateral columns (Nyberg-Hansen and Mascitti, 1964; Petras, 1967). The lateral reticulospinal tract arises in the reticular formation of the medial medulla (Fox, 1970; Valverde, 1962) and its fibers run in the dorsal and lateral aspects of the anterolateral columns (Nyberg-Hansen, 1965; Petras, 1967). Selective spinal cord transections have shown that descending tracts running in the anterolateral columns are sufficient for lordosis (Kow et al., 1977). Conversely, large bilateral transections destroying all anterolateral fibers can eliminate lordosis, showing that descending systems running there are necessary (Kow et al., 1977). This further implicates the lateral vestibulospinal and lateral reticulospinal tracts.

Lesions have shown the contributions of the lateral vestibular nucleus and the nucleus gigantocellularis, the respective sources (Brodal, 1969; Zemlan and Pfaff, 1979; Zemlan et al., 1979) of the lateral vestibulospinal tract and the lateral reticulospinal tract. Damage to the lateral vestibular nucleus produced substantial decrements in lordosis behavior of female rats (Figure 10–3; Modianos and Pfaff, 1976b). In this experiment, in which the first postoperative behavioral tests were conducted weeks after the lesion was made (Modianos and Pfaff, 1976b), relatively small lesions of the nucleus gigantocellularis produced less pronounced but statistically significant lordosis losses. For both lateral vestibular and medullary reticular lesions, the postoperative lordosis quotient was negatively correlated with the percent loss of giant cells in either of these two structures (Figure 10–4). As expected, some lesions of brainstem

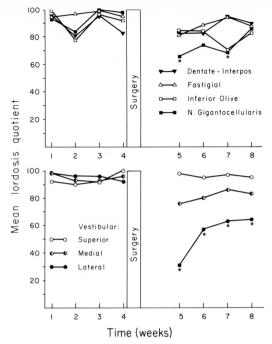

Figure 10–3. Mean lordosis quotients for lesion groups in preoperative and postoperative weekly lordosis reflex tests. *, Significant difference ($p < .025$ in Wilcoxon matched-pairs signed ranks test) between each group's weekly post-operative lordosis quotient and that group's mean preoperative lordosis results. (From Modianos & Pfaff, 1976b)

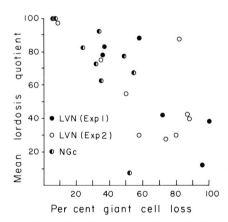

Figure 10–4. Mean postoperative lordosis quotient plotted against percent Dei-ter's cell loss in lateral vestibular nucleus (*LVN*) lesioned rats and percent giant cell loss in nucleus gigantocellularis (*NGc*) lesioned rats. Each point represents data from an individual rat. Correlations between giant cell loss and postoperative lordosis quotient were as follows: for LVN (Exp. 1), $r = -.87$; for LVN (Exp. 2), $r = -.61$; and for nGc, $r = -.70$. (From Modianos & Pfaff, 1976b)

structures in these experiments led to deficits of posture and movement, but these were no statistically related, either within or across groups, to the magnitude of lordosis loss (Modianos and Pfaff, 1976a).

The long postoperative recovery periods allowed in our initial experiments may have permitted significant recovery of function following nucleus gigantocellularis lesions, especially considering that the lesions destroyed only a small portion of the target structure. In a subsequent experiment (Modianos and Pfaff, 1979) female rats were lightly anesthetized with halothane, lesioned, and then tested 4 hours later. Control lesions of the cerebellar cortex or the spinal nucleus of the trigeminal nerve had no effect on the lordosis quotient. Lesions of the nucleus gigantocellularis in the medullary reticular formation or the lateral vestibular nucleus (Figure 10–5) caused pronounced decreases in the lordosis quotient (Figure 10–6). Larger lesions caused lower postopera-

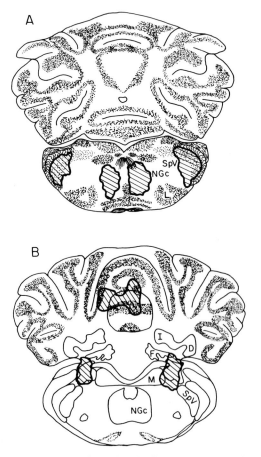

Figure 10–5. A and B. Lesion sites (*hatched areas*). (A) In the nucleus gigantocellularis or (*NGc*), spinal trigeminal nucleus (*SpV*). (B) In the lateral vestibular nucleus or cerebellar cortex. (Data from Modianos & Pfaff, 1979)

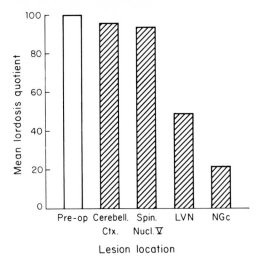

Figure 10–6. Lesions in the lateral vestibular nucleus (*LVN*) or medullary reticular formation (*NGc*) led to significant decreases in lordosis. (From Modianos & Pfaff, 1979)

tive lordosis quotients (Figure 10–7). Under these sensitive experimental procedures (large reticular lesions and short postoperative intervals), the nucleus gigantocellularis appeared to make a much larger contribution to lordosis than in the previous experiment with long postoperative intervals. However, the effect of lateral vestibular nucleus lesions was about the same regardless of the length of the postoperative time. Thus, following subtotal lesions, rats may recover from medullary reticular

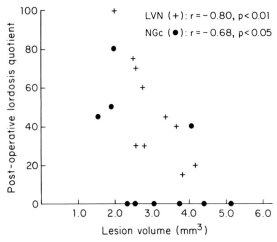

Figure 10–7. Greater lesion volumes in the lateral vestibular nucleus (*LVN*) or medullary reticular formation (*NGc* tended to produce greater postoperative loss of lordosis performance. Each point is the result from an individual rat. (From Modianos & Pfaff, 1979)

lesions more completely or more rapidly than from lateral vestibular lesions. Finally, subsequent lesion experiments showed the dependence of the medullary reticular contribution on experimental conditions (Zemlan, Kow, and Pfaff, 1980a). Deficits in lordosis following lesions of medullary reticulospinal cells, as defined in our laboratory, were larger with larger reticular lesions and shorter postoperative times.

All of these results show that Deiter's neurons in the lateral vestibular nucleus (acting through the lateral vestibulospinal tract) and neurons in the ventromedial medullary reticular formation (acting through the lateral reticulospinal tract) contribute to the descending control of lordosis behavior.

Whereas lateral vestibular lesions interfered with lordosis, electrical stimulation of the lateral vestibular nucleus facilitated it (Modianos and Pfaff, 1975, 1977). In female rats ovariectomized and primed with estrogen, electrical stimulation caused lordosis increases both in tests with manual somatosensory stimulation on the flank and rump–perineal skin regions (Figure 10–8) and in tests where somatosensory stimulation was supplied by the male rat. Unilateral electrical stimulation of the lateral vestibular nucleus often was effective. The magnitude of lordosis facilitation increased with an increased number of pulses per second or increased amperage (Figure 10–9). In some rats, the duration of individual lordosis reflexes was also greatly increased, while in other rats the amount of somatosensory stimulation required for lordosis was reduced.

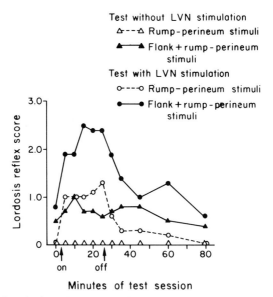

Figure 10–8. Lordosis reflex scores for a female rat before, during, and after electrical stimulation of the lateral vestibular nucleus (*LVN*) and in tests with the same time course, but without LVN stimulation. Note that two types of manual stimulation were used. (From Modianos & Pfaff, 1977)

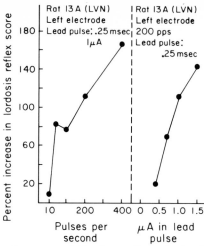

Figure 10–9. Lordosis reflex scores following unilateral stimulation of the lateral vestibular nucleus (*LVN*). *Left-hand side:* all stimulation parameters except pulse frequency were kept constant in this series of tests. *Right-hand side:* all stimulation parameters except amperage in the leading, cathodal pulse were kept constant. (From Modianos & Pfaff, 1977)

Electrical stimulation of the lateral vestibular nucleus did not substitute for estradiol. The stimulation was not effective in facilitating lordosis if the female was completely unreceptive prior to electrical stimulation trials. Parallel to the quantitative correlational analyses of the lesion results (see above), the magnitude of the electrical stimulation effect on lordosis was inversely correlated with the distance of the electrode tip from the center of the lateral vestibular nucleus (Modianos and Pfaff, 1977).

Facilitation of lordosis by pathways from the brainstem to the spinal cord appears to depend on the action of the lateral vestibulospinal tract and the lateral reticulospinal tract.

C.   Electrophysiology of Lateral Vestibulospinal and Lateral Reticulospinal Tracts

1.   Lateral Vestibulospinal Tract: Background

Lateral vestibulospinal fibers tend to terminate on the medial side of the ventral horn, where motoneurons for axial muscles are mainly located (Nyberg-Hansen, 1975). In fact, motoneurons controlling the lateral longissimus dorsi and multifidus muscles, responsible for the vertebral dorsiflexion of lordosis in female rats (Brink, Modianos, and Pfaff, 1979;

Brink and Pfaff, 1979a), are located primarily on the medial and ventro-medial sides of the ventral horn in female rats (Brink, Morrell, and Pfaff, 1979). In a different field of investigation, Lawrence and Kuypers (1968a,b) found that in monkeys interruption of descending pathways whose axons take a ventromedial course (including the lateral vestibulospinal tract) produces severe impairment of axial movements. Very early observations indicated that vestibular lesions are followed by a loss of postural muscle tone (Ewald, 1892).

All of these facts can be summarized by saying that an important function of the lateral vestibulospinal tract is to maintain the tone of axial muscles, including the deep back muscles, which, in female rodents, are important for lordosis. In turn, this physiological characterization fits well with the facilitation of lordosis by electrical stimulation of the lateral vestibular nucleus (Modianos and Pfaff, 1977).

Several neurophysiological characteristics of the lateral vestibulospinal tract are consonant with an important role in lordosis. Its predominant facilitatory effect is on the motoneurons for extensor muscles (V. J. Wilson, 1975a; see also Wilson and Yoshida, 1969; Wilson, Yoshida, and Schor, 1970; Hongo, Kudo, and Tanaka, 1975; ten Bruggencate and Lundberg, 1974; Lund and Pompeiano, 1968; Grillner, Hongo, and Lund, 1970, 1971). Most important for lordosis is the fact that electrical stimulation of the lateral vestibular nucleus can produce excitatory postsynaptic potentials in motoneurons of deep back muscles which cause dorsiflexion of the vertebral column (Wilson et al., 1970). It has also been suggested (ten Bruggencate and Lundberg, 1974) that stimulation of Deiter's cells facilitates extensor motoneurons by excitation of interneurons involved in crossed extensor reflex action evoked from contralateral flexor reflex afferents. In turn, in female rats with complete spinal cord transections, the pattern of drug effects on the crossed extensor reflex (Zemlan et al., 1980b) matches effects on spinal components of lordosis (Kow et al., 1980b). Moreover, the involvement of flexor reflex afferents in the pattern facilitated by the lateral vestibulospinal tract is consistent with lordosis physiology, which may include flexor reflex afferent input (Chapters 3–5).

The organization of Deiter's nucleus itself gives additional clues as to how the lateral vestibulospinal system might participate in lordosis control. Spinovestibular fibers appear to terminate preferentially in the dorsocaudal portion of the lateral vestibular nucleus (Pompeiano and Brodal, 1957). The predominant effect of cutaneous and other somato-sensory input to these Deiter neurons is excitation (Wilson, Kato, Peterson, and Wylie, 1967; Wilson, Kato, Thomas, and Peterson, 1966). The Deiter neurons whose axons project as far as the lumbosacral segments of the spinal cord are located in the same portion of the lateral vestibular nucleus, that is, the dorsocaudal portion (Brodal, 1969; Brodal, Pompeiano, and Walberg, 1962; Nyberg-Hansen, 1975). Thus, in addition to possible tonic effects of lateral vestibulospinal activity on lordosis

mechanisms, another possible lordosis-relevent role for the lateral vestibular nucleus can be construed: cutaneous input due to stimulation by
the male might excite those Deiter neurons whose axons return to
lumbosacral portions of the cord, facilitating motoneurons for muscles
involved in lordosis.

Physiological actions of lateral vestibulospinal fibers are not limited to
effects on or near motoneurons. There is also evidence of effects on
sensory transmission in the spinal cord and on ascending pathways. By
recording potentials from dorsal roots, Cook, Cangiano, and Pompeiano
(1969a,b) have shown that stimulation of the lateral vestibular nucleus
results in negative dorsal root potentials (which correlate with primary
afferent depolarization). Destruction of the vestibular nuclei abolishes
the effect, while transection of either the dorsal columns or the ventromedial columns has no effect on the dorsal root potentials. If the
ventromedial transection includes the medial portion of the anterolateral
columns, the root potentials are abolished.

Therefore, by a process of elimination, we conclude that the lateral
vestibulospinal and perhaps reticulospinal tracts mediate the effect. A
vestibuloreticulospinal link might be considered, since ipsilateral hemisection of the spinal cord only partially depresses dorsal root potentials
evoked from the lateral vestibular nucleus, and the lateral vestibulospinal
tract is an ipsilateral tract (Brodal, 1969). Furthermore, Cook et al.
(1969a,b) showed that the presence of the cerebellum is not required for
obtaining the negative root potentials. Chan and Barnes (1972) reported
that primary afferent depolarization can be obtained from stimulation
points in the medial pontine and medullary reticular formation.

In regard to ascending pathways, it is interesting that the lateral
vestibular nuclei have not been shown to influence transmission ascending through the dorsal or dorsolateral columns, but do influence ascending
information running in the anterolateral columns (reviewed by Pompeiano, 1975). Spinoreticular neurons whose axons ascend in the anterolateral columns receive excitatory influences from the lateral vestibulospinal tract (Holmqvist, Lundberg, and Oscarsson, 1960a,b). Thus, the
pattern of lateral vestibulospinal influences on ascending pathways
matches results on ascending fiber systems in lordosis (Chapter 5): both
sets of results focus on spinoreticular systems in the anterolateral
columns. If lateral vestibulospinal influences in the lumbosacral cord
facilitate ascending systems, which in turn excite Deiter's neurons in the
dorsocaudal lateral vestibular nucleus, it can be seen how rapid postural
adaptations to somatosensory input could be achieved.

Although the strongest effects of the lateral vestibulospinal tract are
on the ipsilateral side of the spinal cord, qualitatively similar effects are
seen on the contralateral side: predominant excitation of extensor and
inhibition of flexor motoneurons (Nyberg-Hansen, 1975; V.J. Wilson,
1975a). Lateral vestibulospinal stimulation can evoke excitatory postsynaptic potentials in both ipsilateral and contralateral extensor motoneurons

(Hongo et al., 1975). The crossed effects are not due to activation of the contralateral vestibulospinal tract by way of crossing fibers of the ipsilateral tract, since transection of the contralateral half of the spinal cord above the level of recording does not abolish the crossed excitation effect. Whether or not some of the stimulation effects might be due to activation of reticulospinal cells is difficult to determine, but recording from the contralateral cord is not affected by a midsagittal transection of the brainstem extending from the lateral vestibular nucleus to the obex (Hongo et al., 1975). The vestibuloreticular interactions demonstrated with neuroanatomical (Ladpli and Brodal, 1968) and physiological (Peterson and Felpel, 1971) techniques indicate that a vestibuloreticulospinal system could cross at a level below the obex. Nevertheless, Hongo et al. (1975) suggest that the contralateral interaction occurs at the spinal level of recording and involves a crossing interneuron. Since the lordosis reflex involves bilaterally symmetrical movements—primarily a bilateral dorsiflexing action on the vertebral column—it makes sense that the lateral vestibulospinal system, shown to be involved in lordosis by lesion and stimulation experiments, has similar actions on both sides of the spinal cord.

Individual axons of the lateral vestibulospinal tract branch to innervate more than one level of the spinal cord (Abzug, Maeda, Peterson, and Wilson, 1974). For instance, antidromic activation of individual lateral vestibulospinal neurons could be obtained both from local branches in the gray matter of cervical or thoracic cord and from the lateral vestibulospinal tract at lumbar levels. Although the branching patterns are not homogenous and unrestricted (Wilson, Uchino, Susswein, and Rapoport, 1976), it appears that information carried by individual vestibulospinal neurons can be passed to a wide variety of spinal cord levels. On the one hand, this places an upper limit on the specificity of information likely to be carried by such neurons. On the other hand, it shows nicely how the lateral vestibulospinal system could participate in lordosis, a reflex that involves vertebral column dorsiflexion from the posterior rump and tailbase all the way forward to the neck.

2.   Lateral (Medullary) Reticulospinal Tract: Background

Reticulospinal axons running in the anterolateral columns to lumbar levels arise primarily from cells in the caudoventral part of the nucleus gigantocellularis in the reticular formation of the medulla (Zemlan et al., 1979; Zemlan and Pfaff, 1979; Peterson, Maunz, Pitts, and Markel, 1975). Transection and lesion experiments cited above suggest that these reticulospinal axons running in more lateral positions through the spinal cord (rather than the ventral columns) are most important for lordosis. Therefore, lordosis should depend on reticulospinal neurons in the caudoventral medulla whose axons run through the anterolateral columns. Indeed, the medullary reticulospinal system may help to carry hypothalamic influences to the spinal cord (Chapter 9).

Magoun and his colleagues showed that electrical stimulation of the ventral part of the medial medullary reticular formation inhibited limb reflexes (Magoun and Rhines, 1946, Schreiner, Lindsley, and Magoun, 1948; Lindsley, Schreiner, and Magoun, 1949). In contrast, electrical stimulation of the pontine reticular formation facilitated limb reflexes (Rhines and Magoun, 1946; Sprague et al., 1948; Lindsley, 1952; Magoun, 1963). Many of these experiments showed bilateral effects of reticular stimulation with similar actions on flexor and extensor reflexes. Later work, including the use of threshold levels of stimulation, uncovered reciprocal effects of reticular stimulation on flexor and extensor reflexes of the legs (Sprague and Chambers, 1954). Reticulospinal axons mediating these effects descend in the anterolateral columns (Niemer and Magoun, 1947). The spinal transections that can abolish these reticulospinal effects appear to be similar in location and size to those that can abolish lordosis (Kow et al., 1977).

Reticulospinal axons are included in the "ventromedial group" of descending systems described by Lawrence and Kuypers (1968a,b) as controlling axial musculature. Brainstem reticular neurons with differing inputs and outputs are interspersed with each other and not arranged according to physiological properties in large, easily recognized nuclei (Eccles, Nicoll, Rantucci, et al., 1976). The synaptic arrangements underlying reticular effects on spinal reflexes are not yet clear. Inputs to reticulospinal neurons have been characterized by means of modern recording techniques (Peterson, Anderson, and Filion, 1974; Peterson, Filion, Felpel, and Abzug, 1975; Peterson and Absug, 1975). Of special interest is the demonstration that neurons deep to the superior colliculus, including laterally situated subtectal neurons, produce excitatory post-synaptic potentials in ipsilateral reticular neurons (Peterson et al., 1974). Cutaneous stimuli also evoke postsynaptic potentials in reticulospinal neurons (Peterson et al., 1974). Reticulospinal neurons in the medulla thus appear to share several physiological properties with likely lordosis mechanisms: they receive a cutaneous input, are involved with descending excitation from subtectal regions, and are involved in the control of axial musculature.

Patterns of postsynaptic potentials in spinal cord motoneurons following reticulospinal activation emphasize the role of this system in the control of axial muscles (Peterson, 1979). Electrical stimulation of the nucleus gigantocellularis leads to monosynaptic excitatory postsynaptic potentials in neck motoneurons on both sides of the cord (Peterson, Pitts, Fukushima, and Mackel, 1978). This shows axial control of a bilateral sort well suited for a response such as lordosis. Ventral nucleus gigantocellularis stimulation can excite back muscle motoneurons mon-osynaptically even under conditions in which limb effects are delayed or weaker (Peterson, Pitts, and Fukushima, 1979). These axial motoneuron effects appear to depend on lateral reticulospinal fibers, already implicated in lordosis.

Like vestibulospinal neurons, individual reticulospinal neurons send branched axons to different levels of the spinal cord (Peterson, Maunz, Pitts, and Mackel, 1975). Individual reticular neurons that can be antidromically activated by stimulation within the gray matter of the cervical spinal cord can also be antidromically stimulated from the lumbar spinal cord. In addition to sending large numbers of axons down the ipsilateral lateral reticulospinal tract, medullary reticular neurons send a few down the contralateral lateral reticulospinal tract (Peterson, Maunz, Pitts, and Mackel, 1975); such axons can participate in the bilateral effects of reticulospinal stimulation on reflexes. The longitudinal branching and bilateral crossing properites of reticulospinal axons are well suited for participation in lordosis control, since lordosis involves dorsiflexion of a large portion of the vertebral column and is bilaterally nearly symmetrical in its appearance.

Physiological experiments with monosynaptic reflexes involving hindlimb motoneuron pools have suggested that some descending effects result from the combined actions of the lateral vestibulospinal and reticulospinal tracts (Hassen and Barnes, 1975); this is also likely to be the case for the control of lordosis.

Thus, transection, lesion, and stimulation data (Sections A and B.2) and electrophysiological properties all indicate that the lateral vestibulospinal and lateral reticulospinal tracts work together in the control of the lordosis reflex. Since no obvious anatomical connections link the hypothalamus or midbrain central gray to the lateral vestibular nucleus, we assume that the lateral vestibulospinal tract does not function as a carrier of descending hypothalamic influences. In contrast, reticulospinal cells in the medullary reticular formation receive descending influences from midbrain structures (central gray and dorsal lateral reticular formation) which in turn receive direct axonal connections from hypothalamic regions involved in lordosis control (Chapter 9). Therefore, we suggest that medullary reticulospinal neurons, operating through the lateral reticulospinal tracts, play an important integrative role in the control of lordosis and, in particular, help to relay descending, hormone-dependent influences from the hypothalamus. Both the lateral vestibulospinal and lateral reticulospinal tracts are known to be involved in the regulation of axial musculature and to have crossed effects similar to their ipsilateral actions. Both of these properties make these tracts suitable for the regulation of lordosis, a vertebral dorsiflexion which is essentially bilaterally symmetrical. Since female rats with complete spinal transections do not perform lordosis (Kow et al., 1977; Pfaff et al., 1972), the net influence of these tracts must be facilitatory for lordosis. Therefore, the net action of the lateral vestibulospinal and lateral reticulospinal tracts must be to increase activity in spinal cord neurons excitatory for lordosis or to inhibit activity in spinal circuits inhibitory for lordosis.

With the HRP technique, cell bodies of reticulospinal neurons can be found in especially great numbers in the ventral caudal part of the medullary reticular formation (Zemlan and Pfaff, 1979; Zemlan et al., 1979). Descending axons from the central gray and dorsal lateral reticular formation of the mesencephalon enter the same region. At first, the emphasis on this part of the medullary reticular formation for lordosis control could seem puzzling because it contains Magoun's (1950) "inhibitory" reticular mechanism, whereas the net reticulospinal effect for lordosis is facilitatory. However, Magoun's studies were on reflexes on the limbs. Electrical stimulation of the ventromedial medullary reticular formation brings locomotion and limb movement to a halt (Magoun, 1950). This is precisely what is needed as part of lordosis facilitation, since the initiation of lordosis in the estrogen-primed female rat requires that she stand still upon cutaneous contact from the male, just prior to active vertebral dorsiflexion (Pfaff and Lewis, 1974). Moreover, the transections of lateral and anterolateral columns needed to disrupt the descending effects of this medullary reticulospinal system (Niemer and Magoun, 1947) are those needed to eliminate lordosis in estrogen-primed female rats (Kow et al., 1977). Therefore, it seems likely that reticulospinal neurons in the ventral and caudal portions of the medullary reticular formation, acting through the anterolateral columns, facilitate lordosis by halting locomotion as well as by facilitating axial reflexes.

3. Electrophysiological Experiments Related to Lordosis

Single units in the nucleus gigantocellularis can respond to cutaneous stimuli on the flanks (Figure 5–5). However, the effective stimuli are of the field unit type (hair movement), which prepares the female rat for lordosis but does not itself trigger the reflex. Even during chronic recording experiments with unanesthetized, freely moving, estrogen-injected female rats (Kow and Pfaff, 1980), medullary reticular units that respond to perineal pressure adequate for triggering lordosis have not been found. It appears that in female rats medullary reticular units do not foster lordosis by virute of rapid strong responses to perineal stimulation, in the manner of a spinobulbospinal reflex. In particular, the units that carry medullary reticular influences to the lumbar spinal cord, the antidromically identified reticulospinal units, have not been shown to respond to lordosis-relevant somatosensory stimuli (Figure 5–6; Kow and Pfaff, 1980). By virtue of behaviorally relevant changes in unit activity over a longer time course and/or responses to preliminary stimulation from the male (for instance, on the flanks), it appears that medullary reticulospinal units *prepare* spinal lordosis reflex circuits for the final (perineal) behavior-triggering stimulus. Such descending effects must eventually register on the motoneurons that cause the execution of lordosis behavior.

The muscles that execute the lordosis response are the lateral longissimus and the transversospinalis system (Chapter 11). Another epaxial muscle is the medial longissimus, which elevates the tailbase. The lateral longissimus and the transversospinalis system are anatomically connected to produce lumbar vertebral dorsiflexion (Brink and Pfaff, 1979a). Their ablation reduces the strength of the lordosis reflex according to the amount of muscle removed (Brink, Modianos, and Pfaff, 1979). Descending influences from the lateral vestibular nucleus and the medullary reticular nucleus gigantocellularis facilitate activity in the motor nerves leading to these muscles (Brink and Pfaff, 1979b, 1980).

The lateral longissimus is a lumbar back muscle innervated by dorsal rami along its length. The medial longissimus, a proximal tail muscle, is innervated by branches from L_6, S_1, and S_2. We recorded electrical activity in the motor nerves for these muscles in urethane-anesthetized female rats (Brink, Pfaff 1979b, 1980). Areas electrically stimulated for the study of inputs and descending influences included the lumbosacral dorsal roots, the medial medullary reticular formation, the lateral vestibular nucleus, the midbrain central gray, and the ventromedial hypothalamus. Electrical stimulation in the lateral vestibular nucleus facilitated motor nerve responses to dorsal root stimulation (Figure 10–10). Trains

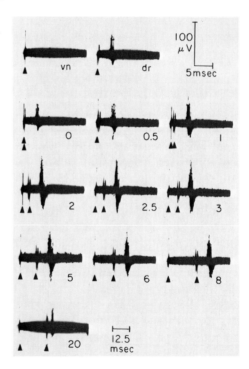

Figure 10–10. Electrical stimulation of the lateral vestibular nucleus facilitated responses of medial longissimus montoneurons to dorsal root stimulation. Stimuli to the vestibular nucleus (*vn*) and dorsal roots (*dr*) alone were set to elicit small or no response. Then they were paired. Conditioning pulses to vn which preceded dr stimulation by 1, 2, 2.5 and 3 msec, for example, greatly facilitated the motor nerve response to dr. (From Brink & Pfaff, 1979b, 1980)

of 5–12 shocks were usually required for facilitation, with optimum condition–test intervals of 2–4 milliseconds. Electrical stimulation of the medial medullary reticular formation also facilitated motor nerve responses to dorsal root stimulation (Figure 10–11). Reticular effects appeared following trains of 1–5 shocks, with condition–test intervals of 0.5–2 milliseconds. Interestingly, electrical stimulation of the central gray of the midbrain had similar facilitating effects (Figure 10–12). Here, conditioning required train lengths of 9–20 shocks, with longer condition–test intervals (5–20 milliseconds). In contrast, electrical stimulation of the ventromedial hypothalamus never facilitated motor nerve activity in these experiments, even with high currents and long trains of hypothalamic stimulation (Table 10–1). Thus, influences from the midbrain central gray, lateral vestibular nucleus, and medial medullary reticular formation excite electrical activity in motor nerves for epaxial back muscles that dorsiflex the vertebral column (Brink and Pfaff, 1979b, 1980). Such influences would facilitate reflex vertebral dorsiflexion in such a way as to promote lordosis.

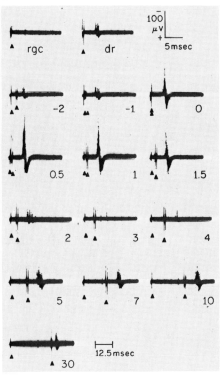

Figure 10–11. Electrical stimulation of the medullary reticular formation facilitated medial longissimus motoneuron response to dorsal root stimulation. Stimuli to reticular formation (*rgc*) and dorsal root (*dr*) were set (top row) to evoke small or no responses. Then (following rows) both were stimulated. Numbers = rgc-dr interval in milliseconds. For example, see large facilitation at rgc-dr interval of 0.5 milliseconds. (From Brink & Pfaff, 1979, 1980)

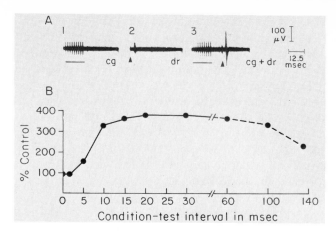

Figure 10–12. Electrical stimulation of the midbrain central gray facilitated medial longissimus motoneuron response to dorsal root stimulation. (From Brink & Pfaff, 1979b, 1980)

Table 10-1. Summary of results of medial longissimus and lateral longissimus nerve recording experiments

Structure Stimulated	Nerve Responses	
	ML	*LL*
Single		
DR	18/18	(8 + 4)/12
PUD	3/6	0/2
LVN	15/15	11/11
RGC	10/11	4/7
VMH	0/9	0/8
Interaction		
LVN/DR	13/14	(5 + 1)/10
RGC/DR	6/10	0/6
VMH/DR	0/9	0/8
LVN + RGC + VM/PUD	0/5	NE

Note. ML, medial longissimus; LL, lateral longissimus; DR, dorsal roots; PUD, pudendal; LVN, lateral vestibular nucleus; RGC, nucleus giganto + cellularis; VMH, ventromedial hypothalamus; NE, not examined.

Data from Brink & Pfaff, 1979b, 1980.

D.   Implications

1.   Specificity of Descending Control

Individual axons of the lateral vestibulospinal tract and lateral reticulo-spinal tract branch to terminate in a variety of different spinal levels. Both of these tracts also have crossed effects similar to their ipsilateral actions. Both of these properties are suited for lordosis control, since the vertebral dorsiflexion of lordosis involves many different levels of the spinal cord and since lordosis is bilaterally symmetrical.

These properties of the lateral vestibulospinal and reticulospinal tracts also place upper limits on the specificity with which these tracts can act. For instance, it seems unlikely that the descending action of fibers in these tracts would specifically facilitate lordosis without affecting other reflex patterns. This lack of perfect specificity is also apparent in the effects of transections and lesions during experiments on lordosis. When spinal columns were transected, it appeared that any portion of the anterolateral columns remaining after transection, as long as it was larger than 25% or 30% of the cross-sectional area of the columns, would support fairly high levels of lordosis behavior (Kow et al., 1977). If any 30% of the anterolateral columns would support the behavior, without regard to which 30%, then the specificity with which individual fibers in those columns act could not be great. Similary, in lesion studies of nuclei giving rise to the lateral vestibulospinal and lateral reticulospinal tracts, the amount of lordosis loss following lesion was a function of the number of giant cells lost, apparently regardless of exactly which giant cells they were (Modianos and Pfaff, 1976b). This finding also probably reflects a relative lack of behavioral specificity in the descending actions of these tracts.

The nature of inputs to reticulospinal neurons also reflects a partial lack of specificity. The cutaneous receptive fields of reticulospinal neurons are usually very large. Moreover, it is likely that a variety of facilitating influences on lordosis can be routed through reticulospinal neurons. For instance, lordosis in estrous female hamsters can be facilitated by olfactory stimuli from the male and by ultrasound (Floody and Pfaff, 1977a,b; Noble, 1972, 1973).

Therefore, if we think of the lordosis response as requiring both precise control of its reflex form and enough amplification to generate sufficient muscular power, we can speak both of a "steering" function and an "acceleratory" function. It now appears that the precise steering control of reflex form must depend largely on spinal circuits, while a relatively gross facilitation of the spinal circuits (amplification, or accel-eration) depends on the combined action of the lateral vestibulospinal and lateral reticulospinal tracts.

Other approaches to the descending control of motor function also allow for a lack of perfect specificity. Midbrain influences on the spinal stepping generator may act, in large part, through a simple increase in postural tone (Mori et al., 1978). A variety of descending influences have been thought to depend upon regulating a single parameter underlying muscle stiffness: the threshold for the stretch reflex (Houk, 1979). Thus, overall, the specific occurrence of lordosis must result from the combination of the descending effects charted above with the exact stimulus pattern arriving at the spinal cord.

Apparently, specificity of a descending influence has not been built into these posture and movement control systems where it is not needed. This economy in the use of neurons on the output side corresponds to the "need to know" principle apparent in the ascending pathways related to lordosis behavior (Chapter 5). We know that it would be impossible to have sets of neurons specifically devoted to every possible behavioral act. The number of possible behavioral acts is too large. The relative lack of behavioral specificity in the descending influences that control lordosis behavior results from the impossibility of a "(one behavioral act): (one neuron set)" formula. Instead, the observed behavioral specificity must lie in the combination of descending influences with specifically keyed stimulus input.

2.   Preparatory Nature of Descending Control

Descending tracts might have either of two modes of action in facilitating lordosis. One is a tonic effect, in which spinal circuits relevant for lordosis would be *prepared* for reflex execution before the onset of the adequate peripheral stimuli. For instance, tonic facilitation might result in a subliminal amount of background activity in motoneuron pools which supply muscles important for lordosis and a corresponding reduction of activity in motoneuron pools for muscles antagonistic to lordosis. Against this prepared background, cutaneous stimuli adequate for lordosis would be able to trigger the behavioral response. A neurophysiological mechanism of this sort could account for the time course of lordosis increases following electrical stimulation of the lateral vestibular nucleus: facilitation due to electrical stimulation often took as long as 5 minutes to reach a peak (Modianos and Pfaff, 1977). If the lateral reticulospinal tract also had a tonic mode of action, as some of the results above indicate, this might reflect the transmission of a tonic, hormone-dependent output from the ventromedial hypothalamus. Another reason for considering tonic modes of action is that conspicuous prelordotic elements of female rodent mating behavior could be involved in providing a tonic increase in the background activity of lordosis-relevant descending systems (Section D.3).

A second mode of action of descending systems could involve spinobulbospinal reflex loops. Although the evidence for reticulospinal neurons is against this as the major mode of action, ascending cutaneous afferents can excite some medullary reticular neurons and vestibulospinal cells (in the dorsocaudal lateral vestibular nucleus). Brainstem neurons receiving lordosis-relevant cutaneous afferents could facilitate the behavior by their projections back down the cord or by the influences on other brainstem neurons. To whatever extent this mechanism operates for either the lateral vestibulospinal or lateral reticulospinal systems, it could still operate in addition to a tonic, preparatory mode of action.

Several lines of evidence favor an important tonic component in the control of lordosis behavior by both the lateral vestibulospinal and lateral reticulospinal tracts. Lordosis is a standing response coupled with vertebral dorsiflexion (Chapter 1). Spinal reflex and muscle organization for this response are not consistent with quick, highly gradated movements. Although while recording from motor nerves we have been able to obtain monosynaptic reflexes (response to electrical stimulation of the dorsal roots), the responses were relatively weak and often required multiple shocks (Brink and Pfaff, 1979b, 1980). In other axial muscles also, the absence or weakness of monosynaptic reflxes was apparent (Abrahams et al., 1978). Many of our lesions and transections affecting lordosis equally affected posture. This was true of spinal cord transections (Kow, Montgomery and Pfaff, 1977). Following subtotal lesions of the nucleus gigantocellularis, the recovery of the lordosis behavior from its lowest performance paralleled the recovery of postural support reflexes and was independent of walking (Zemlan, Kow and Pfaff, 1980a). Responses to adequate cutaneous stimuli were not frequent among cells in the nucleus gigantocellularis and were almost absent in antidromically identified reticulospinal cells (Kow and Pfaff, 1980). All of these facts suggest that the major nucleus gigantocellularis effect is not in the form of a spinobulbospinal reflex, but rather of a slower, preparatory action. This action is in the form of a postural control, rather than control of the distal muscles in a limb.

Extending this idea, we see that the time course of the preparatory action in lordosis-relevant neural circuitry may be reflected in how far anterior in the neuraxis the nerve cells are located. Obviously, the most immediate behaviorally relevant action would be at lumbar spinal cord levels. Preparatory action with a longer time course appears to take place in the lower brainstem. Some components of tonic facilitation may also occur in the central gray of the mesencephalon. Finally, the longest time course of cellular preparation for lordosis behavior must occur in and around the ventromedial nucleus of the hypothalamus, where long-acting estrogenic effects are registered.

3.   Courtship Behaviors Prepare for Lordosis Reflex

Before lordosis, in the vicinity of a male rat, highly receptive female rats well primed with estrogen and progesterone may show an unusual pattern of locomotion (''hopping and darting'') and sudden head movements that result in "ear wiggling." The darting form of locomotion consists of sudden bursts of forward movement followed by sudden stops. The sudden stops promote successful male–female mating encounters (Pfaff et al., 1972, pp. 279–280) (a) by increasing the chance that the male, following from the rear, will bump into the female and (b) by putting the female in a bilaterally balanced posture prepared to support the weight of the male. The sudden darts and stops also leave the female in a state of muscular tension which, although vaguely defined, is known to facilate lordosis (Pfaff et al., 1972). The way in which these courtship behaviors (hopping and darting and ear wiggling) facilitate lordosis behavior can be understood in terms of the electrophysiological features of the lateral vestibulospinal system, which is known to be involved in lordosis.

Hopping and darting are comprised of unusual linear accelerations along the longitudinal and vertical axes. Linear acceleration is a sufficient stimulus for firing primary afferents from the utricle of the labyrinth, and the lateral vestibular nucleus receives utricular afferents (Brodal et al., 1962). Thus, linear acceleration during hopping and darting can stimulate the lateral vestibulospinal system and, in a tonic manner, facilitate lordosis by increasing the background activity in this system.

The "ear wiggling" component of courtship behavior of receptive female rats is a function of rapidly alternating head movements (Beach, 1942). It is now evident from slow-motion movie film analyses of mating encounters that ear wiggling is a result of rapid oscillations of the head around the longitudinal (sagittal horizontal) axis (Modianos and Pfaff, unpublished observations; see Pfaff and Modianos, 1980). Such stimulation strongly excites the anterior and posterior semicircular canals of the labyrinth (Mountcastle, 1974, p. 704), which, in turn, send primary afferent fibers to the lateral vestibular nucleus. Peterson (1970) found that head tilting results in monosynaptic and disynaptic excitatory postsynaptic potentials in many cells in the lateral vestibular nucleus, including those that send efferents to the spinal cord. Labyrinthine stimulation can produce excitatory postsynaptic potentials in extensor motoneurons of the spinal cord (Hassen and Barnes, 1975; Wilson et al., 1970). In particular, the anterior semicircular canals have a special role in exciting those Deiter neurons whose axons travel through the lateral vestibulospinal tract (V.J. Wilson, 1975b). This is especially important for the following reasons: (a) such Deiter neurons are known to have excitatory actions on spinal motoneurons involved in vertebral dorsiflexion; (b) their axons running through the lateral vestibulospinal tract can reach the lumbosacral spinal cord; and (c) the lateral vestibulospinal tract is known to be important for lordosis. In fact, stimulation of the anterior semicircular canals causes a head movement upward (Suzuki and Cohen, 1964), showing how this kind of vestibular stimulation could predispose a female rat toward lordosis.

Female rat courtship behaviors, such as hopping and darting and ear wiggling, display an unusually high state of excitation of musculature facilitated by the lateral vestibulospinal system just prior to lordosis. In turn, vestibular stimulation resulting from these courtship behaviors should lead to an even higher pitch of excitation in the lateral vestibulospinal system and the axial musculature stimulated by it. Thus, these courtship behaviors reveal a positive feedback relationship in the loop including the lateral vestibulospinal system, axial musculature, and vestibular input. The excitation of vestibulospinal and axial muscular systems maintained by this positve feedback does not cause lordosis by itself, but prepares the animal for successful lordosis by maintaining high levels of background activity in lordosis-relevant systems. With a tonically elevated level of activity in those spinal circuits important for lordosis, (i.e. with spinal circuits thus prepared), sensory input from adequate cutaneous stimulation can cause a stronger lordosis reflex.

E.   Summary

The lateral vestibulospinal tract (from the lateral vestibular nucleus) and the lateral reticulospinal tract (from the nucleus gigantocellularis in the ventromedial medullary reticular formation) are the descending pathways that facilitate lordosis (Figure 10–13). Lesions of these systems disrupt

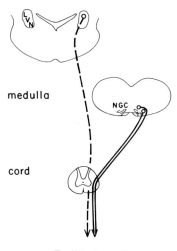

medulla

NGC

cord

Facilitation of
Reflex Vertebral
Dorsiflexion

Figure 10–13. The lateral vestibulospinal tract (from the lateral vestibular nucleus, *LVN*) and lateral reticulospinal tract (from the medullary reticular formation, *NGC*, running in and adjacent to the anterolateral columns of the spinal cord, manage the facilitation of lordosis behavior from the lower brainstem.

the behavior. Electrical stimulation of the lateral vestibular nucleus facilitates it. The electrophysiological properties of both the lateral vestibulospinal and reticulospinal tracts are well suited to their roles in lordosis: they control axial muscle motoneurons, they branch at different vertebral levels, and they act bilaterally. They help in part to prepare spinal circuits for the occurrence of lordosis; for example, the lateral vestibulospinal tract elevates postural tone. The lateral reticulospinal system helps to relay hormone-dependent hypothalamic signals that have been transmitted via the midbrain central gray. The specificity of action of these descending pathways depends on the combination of their influences with specific patterns of cutaneous input.

Chapter 11

Motoneurons and Response Execution

Influences descending from the brainstem to the spinal cord, if they are to affect behavior, eventually must register in the activity of relevant motoneurons. We proceed to discover how this occurs by working our way in from the form of the behavioral response itself to the spinal neural mechanisms that determine that form. Precise descriptions of the behavioral response provide the platform from which studies of the responsible muscles can be launched (Section B); in turn, using those muscle nerves, the responsible motoneurons can then be located and studied with anatomical and electrophysiological techniques (Sections C and D).

A. Response Execution

Lordosis is a standing response marked by an extreme vertebral dorsiflexion. It has the effect of exposing the perineal region to pelvic thrusts from the male, thus allowing fertilization. Precise behavioral descriptions, as summarized in Chapter 1, Section D, have been based on high-speed film analyses (Pfaff and Lewis, 1974; Pfaff et al., 1972) and X-ray cinematography (Pfaff et al., 1978).

Lordosis behavior is distinguished from other responses primarily by the vertebral dorsiflexion. The rump and tailbase are raised, the thorax depressed, and the head elevated (Figure 11–1). Forces that produce this posture have been proven to act on the vertebral column itself (Chapter 1). Therefore, we searched for axial muscles—deep back muscles acting on the vertebral column—that provide the physical basis for lordosis behavior.

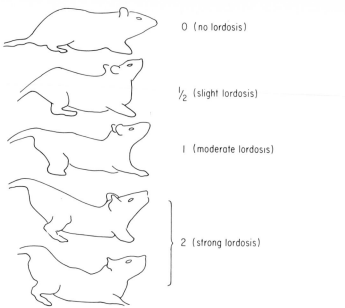

Figure 11–1. Drawings traced from single frames of films of rat mating encounters that illustrate lordosis behavior and show the reflex strength measure used in muscle ablation experiments. (From Brink, Modianos, & Pfaff, 1979)

B. Muscles

Which muscles are competent to execute the rump elevation of lordosis? The anatomy of the vertebral muscles of the back and tail of the rat, including the dorsal and ventral vertebral muscles, must be examined

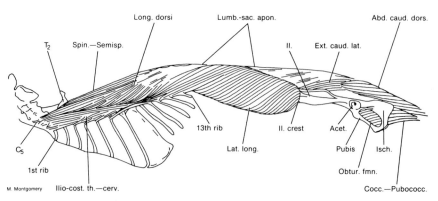

Figure 11–2. Side view of deep vertebral muscles of the albino Norway rat. Muscle has been cleared from the obturator foramen to show the deep-lying coccygeus and pubococcygeus fibers. Extensor caudae lateralis fibers are seen through the thin fascia that separates this muscle from abductor caudae dorsalis. *Lat. long.,* lateral longissimus. (From Brink & Pfaff, 1979a)

(Brink and Pfaff, 1979a). Among the epaxial muscles, the transversospinalis system, the longissimus system, and the iliocostalis system are distinguished. It is clear that the lumbar epaxial muscles are primarily responsible for the rump and tailbase elevation of lordosis. In particular, the lateral longissimus and the lumbar transversospinalis muscles seem anatomically best suited to produce the lumbosacral dorsiflexion of the rump elevation. Both are trunk muscles and are connected such that, dorsiflexion results from bilateral contraction, (Figures 11–2 and 11–3).

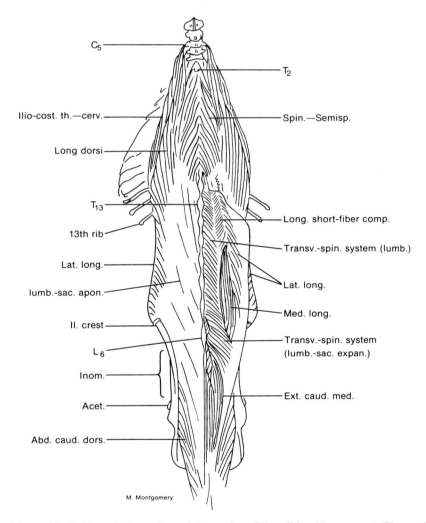

Figure 11–3. Dorsal view of epaxial muscles of the albino Norway rat. The neck is tilted upward such that the cervical vertebrae appear shortened. On the right, the lumbosacral aponeurosis has been cut and deflected laterally to reveal underlying muscles, including fibers of the lateral longissimus *(Lat. long.)* taking origin from the medial face of the aponeurosis. (From Brink & Pfaff, 1979a)

In fact, bilateral electrical stimulation of lumbar transversospinalis muscles during anatomical experiments produces local dorsiflexion of the vertebral column. Bilateral electrical stimulation of the lateral longissimus, with high enough current, yields a strong dorsiflexion including obvious rump elevation.

When lateral longissimus or lumbar transversospinalis muscles are ablated, the strength of the lordosis response declines, roughly according to the amount of muscle removed (Brink, Modianos, and Pfaff, 1979). For example, during tests in which lordosis was assayed by the female's response to stimulation from the male rat, bilateral removal of the lateral longissimus led to a marked decline in response strength, which then recovered slightly over a period of days (Figure 11–4). Subsequent additional removal of lumbar transversospinalis muscles virtually abolished lordosis behavior (Figure 11–4). Identical effects were seen in tests in which lordoses were elicited by artificial cutaneous stimulation (Figure 11–5). Initial removal of the lateral longissimus caused lordosis virtually

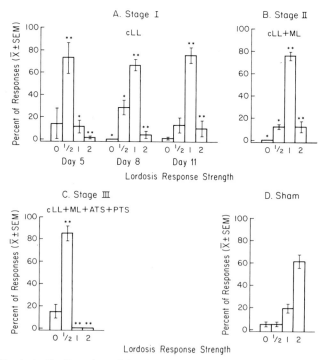

Figure 11–4 A–D. Results of lordosis tests with stimulation by male rats (lordosis scale 0–2 as in Figure 11–1). (A) "Complete lateral longissimus" muscle ablations (*cLL*) significantly weakened lordosis strength. (B) After some recovery from this (graph A, Day 11), medial longissimus (*ML*) ablations did not add to the deficit. (C) Added ablations of anterior and posterior transversospinalis muscles (*ATS + PTS*) rendered lordosis barely detectable. (D) Sham-operated controls. (From Brink, Modianos, & Pfaff, 1979)

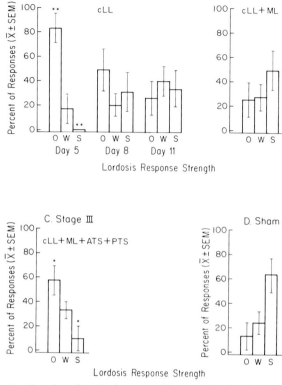

Figure 11–5 A–D. Results of lordosis tests with manual stimulation, *0*, no reflex; *W*, weak; *S*, strong. (A) "Complete lateral longissimus" ablations (*cLL*) virtually abolished the lordosis response (Day 5), which then recovered (Day 11). (B) Added medial longissimus (*ML*) ablations did not cause further loss. (C) Added anterior and posterior transversospinalis muscle ablations (*ATS* + *PTS*) then significantly weakened the reflex. (D) Sham-operated controls. (From Brink, Modianos, & Pfaff, 1979)

to disappear, followed days later by a partial reappearance. Then, additional removal of transversospinalis muscles just about abolished the response (Figure 11–5). As shown by electromyographic recordings, lateral longissimus muscle fibers really are active during initiation of the lordosis response (Figure 11–6; Schwartz-Giblin and Pfaff, in preparation). Thus, these muscles are active and essential during lordosis behavior.

In summary, the lumbar epaxial muscles, lateral longissimus, and transversospinalis execute the rump elevation (the most critical portion) of lordosis behavior. They are appropriately anatomically connected to perform this action, they are active during the response, their electrical stimulation produces lordosislike movements, and their removal destroys the response.

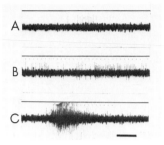

Figure 11–6. Electromyogram recorded from the lateral longissimus during a lordosis reflex elicited by manual stimulation. A. Spontaneous muscle activity recorded during the control period immediately preceding manual stimulation. B. Motor units evoked by bilateral stroking of flanks. C. Strong discharge recorded during the lordosis evoked by pressure applied to the perineum a couple of seconds following flank stimulation. Pressure was maintained until the end of the signal marks seen on the upper trace. Time calibration: 500 milliseconds. (From Schwartz-Giblin & Pfaff, in preparation.)

C.   Motoneurons: Location

Identification of the muscles and motor nerves involved in lordosis enabled us to localize the motoneuron cell bodies involved. One method used was HRP injections in individual lumbar epaxial muscles of female rats (Brink, Morrell, and Pfaff, 1979). Following injection of HRP into the lateral longissimus, HRP-labeled motoneuron cell bodies were found forming a continuous string of cells on the medial side of the ventral horn of the spinal cord, stretching from the posterior half of the lumbar enlargement through and anterior to the enlargement (Figure 11–7). After HRP injection into anteriorly placed transversospinalis muscles, labeled motoneuron cell bodies were seen around the anterior border of the lumbar enlargement and on the medial side and in the ventromedial corner of the ventral horn (Figure 11–8). Following injection into transversospinalis muscles at midlumbar levels, labeled cells formed a string on the medial side of the ventral horn stretching through the enlargement itself and including some cells anterior to the enlargement (Figure 11–9). After HRP injections into posteriorly placed transverso-spinalis muscles, HRP-labeled motoneuron cell bodies were generally found in the ventromedial portion of the ventral horn, from posterior to the lumbar enlargement through to the anterior part of the enlargement (Figure 11–10).

Another method used for localizing motoneuron cell bodies was to track through the spinal cord scanning for sites at which electrical microstimulation produced visible twitches of transversospinalis or me-dial longissimus muscles (Brink, Morrell, and Pfaff, 1979). The locations of sites in the ventral horn that produced twitches of these muscles with

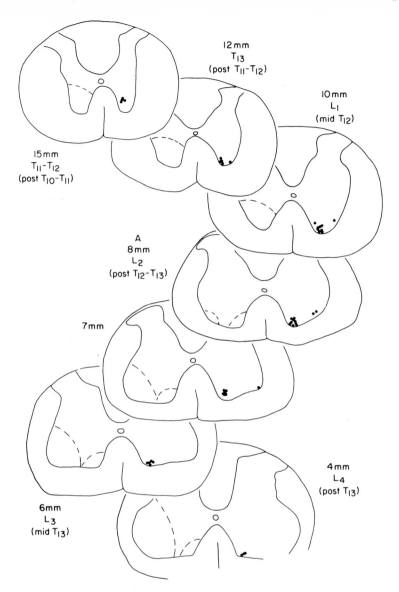

12 mm
T₁₃
(post T₁₁-T₁₂)

10 mm
L₁
(mid T₁₂)

15 mm
T₁₁-T₁₂
(post T₁₀-T₁₁)

A
8 mm
L₂
(post T₁₂-T₁₃)

7 mm

4 mm
L₄
(post T₁₃)

6 mm
L₃
(mid T₁₃)

Figure 11–7. Location of HRP-labeled cells '(*dots*) following injection of HRP into the lateral longissimus. *A* is the anterior boundary of lumbar enlargement. (From Brink, Morrell, & Pfaff, 1979)

the lowest threshold currents were the same as those identified using HRP.

Third, we also localized lumbar epaxial motoneuron cell bodies by extracellular recording of antidromic stimulation in the spinal cord, with dye deposition at the single unit recording site (Brink and Pfaff, 1979b,

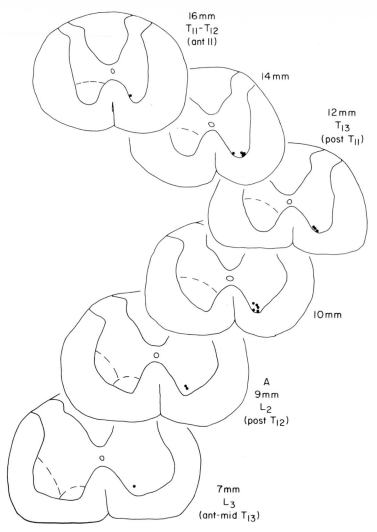

Figure 11–8. Location of HRP-labeled cells (*dots*) following injection of HRP into anterior transversospinalis muscles at the L_3–L_5 level. *A* is the anterior boundary of lumbar enlargement. (From Brink, Morrell, & Pfaff, 1979)

1980). Antidromic single unit potentials (Figure 11–11) were recorded for lateral longissimus motoneurons on the medial side of the ventral horn (Figure 11–12). Those few transversospinalis motoneuron cell bodies encountered were found in the same place.

In summary, lateral longissimus and transversospinalis motoneurons, localized by HRP, microstimulation, or antidromic identification, lie along the medial side of the ventral horn, in and just anterior to the lumbar enlargement.

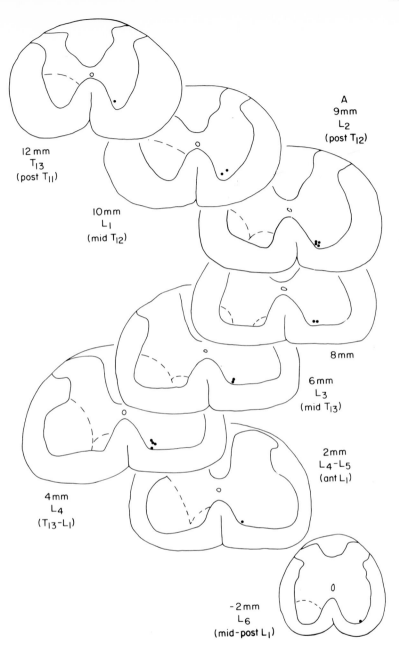

Figure 11–9. Locations of HRP-labeled cells (*dots*) following injection of HRP into middle transversospinalis muscles from anterior L_5 to mid-S_1 levels. *A* is the anterior boundary of lumbar enlargement. (Data from Brink, Morrell, & Pfaff, 1979)

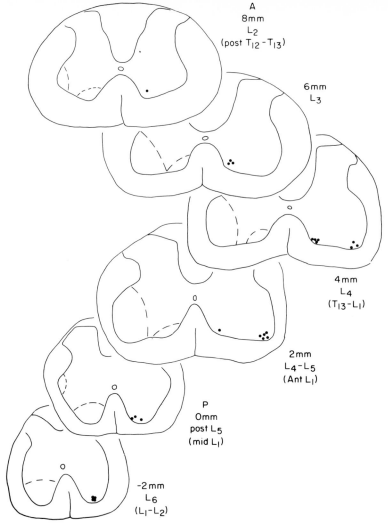

Figure 11–10. Location of HRP-labeled cells (*dots*) following injection of HRP into posterior transversospinalis muscles at the L_5 to posterior S_1 or to anterior S_2 level. *A* is the anterior boundary and *B* is the posterior boundary of lumbar enlargement. (From Brink, Morrell, & Pfaff, 1979)

D. Motoneurons: Physiology

We recorded electrical activity from appropriate motor nerves in order to study dorsal root stimulation responses by motoneurons for lumbar epaxial muscles (Brink and Pfaff, 1979b, 1980). Electrical stimulation of appropriate dorsal roots usually led to a short latency compound action potential on lateral longissimus or medial longissimus nerves. However, to bring out these responses, at least double shocks to the dorsal roots were required. The latencies to motor nerve responses, measured at stimulus intensities just above threshold for evoking the response, were short enough, and, as stimulus strength was increased, stable enough to indicate that these short latency segmental responses probably represent monosynaptic reflexes. For some lateral longissimus nerves, however, stable responses to dorsal root stimulation could not be obtained, even after repeated attempts under various conditions. Thus, while monosynaptic responses on these motor nerves could be recorded, on the whole they were present less frequently and were weaker than expected (Brink and Pfaff, 1979b, 1980). Similarly weak monosynaptic reflexes have been noted for another type of axial muscle—neck muscles in the cat (Abrahams and Rose, 1978).

These results differ from those expected for limb muscle motoneurons. Correspondingly, greater influences from excitatory descending systems would be expected to control these axial muscle motoneurons. Indeed, excitation from the lateral vestibular nucleus and the medullary reticular formation was shown (Chapter 10) to facilitate activity in the types of axial motoneurons relevant for lordosis. Excitatory postsynaptic potentials in axial motoneurons following medullary reticular electrical stimulation indicated direct facilitation (Chapter 10) of these motoneurons by this descending system. Other work (Chapter 10) suggested that interneurons are involved in some descending effects of the lateral vestibulospinal and lateral reticulospinal systems. The parameters of motoneuron–muscle dynamics most closely controlled by lateral vestibular and

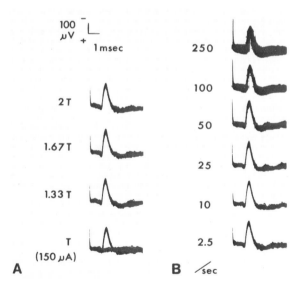

Figure 11–11. Antidromic identification of a medial longissimus motoneuron, showing stability of its antidromic potential across amplitude and frequency of stimulation. (Data from Brink & Pfaff, 1979b, 1980)

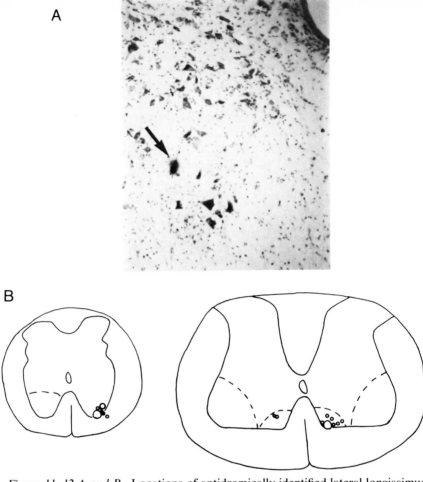

Figure 11–12 A and B. Locations of antidromically identified lateral longissimus (*LL*), and transversospinalis (*TS*) neurons. (A) Photomicrograph of a dye spot (arrow) at the site of one recorded antidromic potential. (B) Maps on spinal cord drawings of several dye spots locating motoneurons for LL (right side of sections) and TS (left side). (Data from Brink & Pfaff, 1979, 1980)

lateral reticular influences (for instance, "muscle stiffness" and the threshold for the stretch reflex; Houk, 1979) remain to be determined.

E.   Summary

The deep back muscles, the lateral longissimus and transversospinalis muscles, execute the vertebral dorsiflexion of lordosis (Figure 11–13). Thus, these muscles are responsible for the rump elevation, the most crucial component, of lordosis behavior. They are connected so as to be

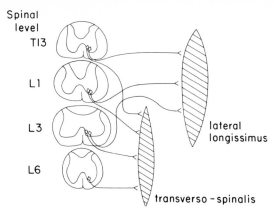

Figure 11–13. Schematic representation of final common pathway for lordosis.

anatomically competent to execute this response, and they are electrically active during the initiation of lordosis. Bilateral electrical stimulation of the lateral longissimus or transversospinalis muscles produces vertebral dorsiflexion. Ablation of these muscles reduces lordosis strength.

The motoneurons for the lateral longissimus and transversospinalis muscles lie on the medial and ventral borders of the ventral horn. They may be found at spinal levels receiving dorsal roots from T_{12} through S_1 (just anterior to, in, and just posterior to the lumbar enlargement).

The monosynaptic reflex for these axial motoneurons appears to be weaker than would be expected for limb muscle motoneurons. Lateral longissimus and transversospinalis motoneurons must receive descending excitatory influences via the lateral vestibulospinal and lateral reticulospinal tracts (Chapter 10). The branches in these descending axons allow axial motoneurons at various levels, on both sides of the spinal cord, to receive descending excitatory influences. The net result of facilitating electrical activity in lateral longissimus and transversospinalis motoneurons in female rats is promotion of the reflex vertebral dorsiflexion of lordosis behavior.

Part 4

Building on this Paradigm

Chapter 12

Logical and Heuristic Developments

A. Introduction

With large parts of the neural circuitry for lordosis behavior determined, we can look for opportunities to generalize. In several cases these facts speak to issues longstanding in the neural control of behavior; in other cases new concepts may be induced. Some principles of operation arise from the input (ascending) side of the lordosis behavior circuit (Sections B and C); other features have more to do with the middle of the circuit (Sections D and F); and still others are related to motor control on the output side of the circuit (Sections G and H). These principles may be considered in relation to the neural control of other behavior patterns.

B. Economy in the Use of Ascending Sensory Information: The "Need to Know" Principle

1. Limited and Selective Distribution of Sensory Information

The most complete and precise forms of sensory information signal the existence of a stimulus and its exact location, time, and form. The very fact of a response by a nerve cell shows recognition that a stimulus event occurred. The size of the receptive field of the nerve cell limits the precision with which the nerve cell can signal exactly where the stimulus occurred. How closely does the nerve cell's response follow the stimulus in time? Latency (and its constancy), duration of response, and afterdischarge are the features that limit the nerve cell's information about when the stimulus occurred. Finally, the type of stimulus that occurred—its

form of energy and the nature of its impingement on the body surface —
is signaled in the modality of response by the nerve cell. For example,
among somatosensory stimuli, the nerve cell might or might not be
specific for pressure, hair deflection, pain, temperature change, etc.

At several points in the neural circuit for lordosis behavior it is
obvious that not all sensory information is transferred (Chapter 5).
Sometimes there is a loss of precision in the sensory information
described above. At other times, there is a simple loss of responsivity
(for instance, in the hypothalamus). For example, in the spinal cord and
brainstem, not all of the stimulus information about space is used: the
exact location of the stimulus on the skin is not necessarily signaled.
Receptive fields become much larger as one goes from the primary
sensory neurons to the relevant interneurons in the spinal cord. In turn,
relevant somatosensory information that reaches the brainstem is even
grosser. Nerve cells in portions of the midbrain relevant for lordosis
behavior have very large receptive fields (Malsbury et al., 1972; Sakuma
and Pfaff, 1980d). The activity of a significant portion of the nerve cells
in the brainstem that controls lordosis does not reflect the exact time of
stimulus application. Indeed, many of these cells seem to be devoted to
longer term changes that prepare the way for adequate response to later
stimulus application. Indeed, some cells in the circuit show no recognition
of the existence of an important stimulus. Nerve cells in the medial
hypothalamus, in regions known to be involved in lordosis control, may
not respond to somatosensory input at all.

On the positive side, loss of stimulus information may actually serve
an integrative function. The increasing size of receptive fields along the
lordosis behavior circuit proves convergence of information (Section C).
This provides a mechanism for the summation of stimuli in the determination of lordosis behavior (Chapter 2).

On the other hand, the distribution of sensory information in lordosis
behavior circuitry has obvious limitations in scope and precision. It is as
though the question had been asked: "What does the nerve cell *need to
know* to do its particular job?" If it needs a certain amount and form of
sensory information to play its role, it gets it; if not, it gets less complete
or less precise sensory input, or no sensory input at all. This reflects a
great economy in the use of nerve cell signaling capacity. If sensory input
to a given nerve cell is not needed, there is none. In the terminology of
spy books about national intelligence agencies, a "need to know"
principle seems to be operating. In spy agencies, the purpose is to
increase security. In the nervous system, application of the "need to
know" principle prevents waste and confusion.

2.   Permitting Neural Plasticity

In order to demonstrate a corollary of the above principle we contrast
stable, stimulus-bound systems with more labile systems that permit
learning and other alterations. In lordosis behavior circuitry, cells that

most faithfully represent stimulus information are found anatomically closest to the stimulus. These nerve cells, at spinal cord segmental levels closest to lordosis-relevent sensory input and motor output, are subject to great stimulus control. From the point of view of lordosis circuit operation, these cells have great stability. In contrast, in upper portions of the circuit, sensory information is less dominant. Analogous portions of other behavior control circuits include not only the reticular formation of the brainstem, but also the cerebral cortex. These portions of behavior control circuitry can be pictured as being relatively free from stimulus control. In that sense, they are labile. This lability is a precondition for neural plasticity.

C.   Additions and Interactions of Behavioral Causes by Nerve Cells: Analogy to "Switching Circuits" and "Threshold Logic"

1.   Additions: The Role of Convergence

In some cases stimuli must be summated across receptor to achieve a given behavior; in order to explain the sensory summation effects that have been reported (Chapter 2), we must conclude this is true for lordosis behavior. Adequate pressure stimuli on three locations of skin were always more effective for triggering lordosis than stimuli covering only two locations (Table 2–1). For achieving a given degree of lordosis performance, less cutaneous pressure was required if the stimulus covered a greater area (Figure 2–4). In female hamsters, as in rats, mechanical stimulation of the skin over a greater area could be summated to trigger a longer or stronger lordosis response (Kow et al., 1976).

In the sensory pathway for lordosis behavior, stimulus information converges from neuron to neuron (Chapter 4). For instance, during recording from primary sensory units in the dorsal root ganglion, few units responding to more than one modality were observed (Kow and Pfaff, 1979). Cutaneous modality information converges, however, on nerve cells in the spinal gray: many units there responded both to hair movement and skin deformation, and other units responded to other combinations of cutaneous stimuli (Kow et al., 1980a). Convergence is also proven by the increases in receptive field size from one level of sensory neuron to the next (Kow and Pfaff, 1979; Kow et al., 1980a). For example, among units responding selectively to pressure, the average receptive field area for spinal interneurons was 61 times as great as that for primary sensory units. In turn, many brainstem units that respond to cutaneous stimuli have receptive fields that cover large portions of the body (Malsbury et al., 1972; Sakuma and Pfaff, 1980d). The skin area required to be stimulated to trigger lordosis is greater than that covered by the receptive field of any spinal interneuron recorded thus far (Kow et al., 1979; Pfaff et al., 1977); therefore, further convergence must occur at a level beyond these interneurons.

Convergence of sensory information onto a small number of neurons is probably the mechanism of the behavioral summation observed. Individual stimulation of receptors, leading to individual activation of primary sensory units, has no behavioral effect. However, simultaneous stimulation of large numbers of receptors, activating a large number of primary sensory units whose outputs converge on spinal interneurons, can trigger female reproductive behavior.

The concept of convergence of neuronal activity as a mechanism of behavioral summation is in agreement with the other theoretical ideas presented here. The combination of particular sensory inputs without preservation of their individual identities is part of the economic use of ascending sensory information. Where convergence is adequate, the postsynaptic neuron does not "need to know" individual receptor identity. In turn, the postsynaptic nerve cell must have a high enough threshold for firing such that the convergence of adequate numbers of primary units is required for its activation. Combined stimulation has the power to drive that type of postsynaptic interneuron, which then must be well placed to assist in driving lordosis motoneurons. This type of setup submits easily to description by threshold logic, as introduced briefly below. Viewed nerve cell by nerve cell, as revealed in our recordings, or according to a description by theshold logic, these phenomena explain summation across receptors in the activation of lordosis behavior.

2. Interactions

a. Stimulus–stimulus. Summations, as described in Chapter 2 and above, are special cases of stimulus–stimulus interactions; the stimuli involved are applied simultaneously or almost so. In other cases, effects of prior stimulation can interact with the effects of the final set of stimuli either to facilitate or to inhibit the lordosis response (reviewed by Kow and Pfaff 1977). An example of a sequential (as opposed to simultaneous) interaction that spans the smallest amount of time would be the facilitation of lordosis response to perineal pressure by flank stimulation immediately preceding it (Pfaff et al., 1977). Over a longer time course, previous interactions with males can facilitate lordosis in female hamsters (Manogue et al., 1980a). Similarly, olfactory stimuli from male hamsters can strengthen a later lordosis response in females (Noble, 1972, 1973). Ultrasound, intended to mimic the auditory signals a female hamster can receive from a male, can strengthen and lengthen the eventual lordosis response to cutaneous input (Floody and Pfaff, 1977a,b).

b. Hormone–stimulus interactions. The most obvious form of interaction occurs when the application of relevant steroid hormones increases the likelihood that a given set of stimuli will lead to a behavioral response. Estrogen or estrogen plus progesterone increases the strength of the lordosis response to a given relevant cutaneous stimulus. Estrogen or estrogen plus progesterone decreases the stimulus strength required for triggering a given amplitude of lordosis response (Diakow et al., 1973; Pfaff et al., 1977). Quantitative measurement of pressure stimulation for triggering lordosis shows this type of interaction most graphically (Kow et al., 1979; Figure 2–5).

In this form of interaction estrogen can be said to increase the strength of the throughput from the relevant cutaneous receptors to lordosis response mechanisms. In fact, this comprises an input–output definition of the estrogen effect.

c. Hormone–hormone interactions. Within fixed stimulus and response strengths and appropriate dose ranges, estrogen and progesterone can substitute for each other in promoting lordosis behavior. If the dose and length of estrogen application are increased, progesterone is not required (Davidson et al., 1968; Pfaff, 1970b). If progesterone is administered, a reduced dose of estrogen is required to produce a given level of lordosis behavior with constant stimulus strength (Diakow et al., 1973; Pfaff et al., 1977).

d. Summary. Thus, among the causal factors that can interact to produce lordosis behavior, we include cutaneous stimulus area, strength of cutaneous pressure (on relevant skin locations), and (at appropriate doses) estrogen dose and progesterone dose. Within the relevant dynamic ranges, an increase in any of these causal factors will increase the strength of lordosis behavior. Correspondingly, if the level of one of these causal factors is low, an increase in another can compensate for it.

3. Formal Descriptions of Behavioral Mechanisms: The Nervous System Can Be Logical

As our knowledge of the neural mechanisms underlying a particular mammalian behavior pattern grows, it becomes important to be able to state our systematic results and hypotheses precisely. In turn, precise statements require a formal language. It is not obvious which formal language will be most helpful for summarizing our knowledge of behaviorally relevant circuitry in the mammalian nervous system and for generating new knowledge of this sort. For example, calculus is supremely useful for the discussion of motion in physics, but may be much too limited to be useful in describing the nervous system. Probably, different formal languages will be optimal for describing different aspects of neural action. Description of the decay of an excitatory postsynaptic potential over distance may indeed require calculus. However, description of the flow of information around a neural circuit and the decisions made thereby requires a clarification of network properties that is probably best accomplished by a system of formal logic. A language that encompasses "switching algebra" would be helpful. Happily, such descriptions can foster computer modeling of neural mechanisms for behavior.

Threshold logic exemplifies the type of system and element description which may be useful. Threshold logic deals with networks composed of threshold elements (Dertouzos, 1965). A threshold element has an output of 0 or 1, and receives any number of inputs that can have the value of 0 or 1. For a given threshold element, the value of any individual input is multiplied by a number called the weight (for that element). Each element has a threshold. Within any unit of time, the output of that threshold element is 1 if and only if the sum of the weighted inputs at that time equals or exceeds the threshold. Otherwise, the output of that threshold element at that time is 0. Threshold elements resemble neurons in at least two respects. The confluence of inputs with weighted sums resembles the many inputs into a nerve cell, physiologically effectively weighted according to the size of their postsynaptic potential contributions at or near the axon hillock. Then, the presence or absence of an action potential generated to head down the axon represents a binary output.

At a systems (network) level of description, threshold logic can be used to describe how circuits switch from one state to another (Hill and Peterson, 1974; Kohavi, 1978). More generally, by means of this logic networks can be synthesized to accomplish certain logical functions. This technique could be important for the description of certain neural mechanisms for behavior: it may be used to explain why a behavioral response does or does not occur under well-established conditions.

Neural mechanisms that manage the addition and interaction of behavioral influences can be described in terms of the adition of weighted inputs whose sum may or may not reach threshold for a given threshold element. For example, if threshold elements represent neurons in sensory pathways for lordosis, then the convergence of sensory information, responsible for the behavioral effects of stimulus summation, would be represented by converging inputs with appropriate weights. The effects of interaction of a steroid hormone with sensory stimuli for reproductive behavior can be depicted by threshold elements standing for hormone-sensitive nerve cells, and the hormone influence itself could be described either as an input with a large weight or as an alteration of the threshold itself.

Using computers to employ threshold logic in the formal description of neural circuitry for reproductive behavior, we expect to be able to generate quantitative predictions which we then can test using electro-physiological methods.

D. Motivation: A Neural Mechanism for Sex Drive

Suppose an organism does not make a given response to a particular stimulus in particular surroundings, but a short time later (without any maturational changes) the same organism does respond in the given way to exactly the same stimulus in exactly the same surroundings. How do we explain the change from absence of response to presence of response? It is not due to a change in the stimulus, a change in context, or long-term changes such as growth. Change in a well-defined response to a fixed stimulus defines a change in *motivation*. The change in motivational state is taken to explain the change in observed behavior. In turn, it is of great interest to provide a physiological explanation of changes in motivational state.

The nature of the neural circuitry for lordosis behavior and the estrogen effects on it described in this book can provide an explanation for a change in motivational state. The input–output concept of the estrogen effect (Chapter 2) is that estrogen increases the strength of the functional connection from cutaneous pressure stimuli on the relevant skin areas in the female rodent to the motor neurons for the deep back musculature which executes lordosis behavior. In fact, this is one example of a stimulus–hormone interaction in the nervous system (Section C).

The physiological description of this motivational effect of estrogen is as follows. Estrogen arrives at nerve cells in and around the ventrolateral portion of the ventromedial nucleus of the hypothalamus and in the preoptic area. Receptors in the cytoplasm and then in the nucleus of those cells concentrate the hormone. As a result, estrogen increases the biosynthetic capacity and electrical excitability of cells in and around the ventromedial nucleus of the hypothalamus. Through their connections to the mesencephalon, these nerve cells prepare brainstem circuitry for lordosis to occur, given adequate cutaneous stimulus input. In the medial preoptic area, estrogen decreases electrical excitability. Since the net effect of those cells is to decrease the occurrence of lordosis, by decreasing their activity estrogen enhances the behavioral response. The motivational effects of these hypothalamic and medial preoptic neurons are read out to mesencephalic neurons in and around the central gray. These mesencephalic neurons control lordosis partly by virtue of their responses to lordosis-relevant ascending input, but mainly by their hormone-dependent output to the medullary reticular formation. In turn, medullary reticulospinal cells (supplemented by lateral vestibulospinal influences) increase the excitability of spinal segmental circuits which execute lordosis behavior: a response to cutaneous pressure stimuli on the relevant skin areas with a vertebral dorsiflexion managed by lateral longissimus and transversospinalis muscles.

This brief description of a physiological mechanism for a motivational change comprises a brief restatement of the lordosis circuitry and estrogen effects upon it which are set forth in the rest of this book, with estrogen viewed as a motivational variable.

Many motivational systems include evidence of "need" on the part of the motivated organism, usually displayed by approach responses. For female reproductive behavior in rodents, the main motivational change explained thus far is the actual occurrence of lordosis behavior. However, mating in female rodents also includes approach ("appetitive") responses. Female rats will perform arbitrarily chosen responses in order to gain access to male rats (Bermant and Westbrook, 1966). The male rats have "incentive" value. Moreover, female rats will cross grids and barriers to approach male rats (Meyerson and Lindstrom, 1973). In fact, their readiness to do so is increased by estrogen. Thus, one index of sex drive in female rodents is the actual occurrence of lordosis behavior, given adequate stimulus input. Sex drive can also be measured, however, by the readiness to seek the male.

The completeness of the lordosis circuitry described to date, the progress in explaining the effects of estrogen on it, and the use of the estrogen effect in explaining a motivational change shows that B. F. Skinner (1953) was wrong in saying that "a drive (or motivation) is not a physiological state." He wanted to prevent false explanations of behavior and the misuse of the idea of motivation as a free explanatory parameter in the absence of adequate behavioral analysis. He did not think that we would have knowledge about neural circuitry and changing internal states of an organism such that treatment of motivation as a physiological variable would have predictive value. However, by showing how neural circuitry for lordosis produces a mating behavior response, by knowing that increased estrogen levels increase the likelihood and strength of that response, and, finally, by describing the impact of estrogen on the behavior-relevant circuitry, we bring the analysis of the physiology of motivation to a new plateau. By imposing experimental endocrine changes and by observing natural estrous states we have determined the changes in estrogen levels. From that information we can predict changes in mating behavior. We have discovered where in the central nervous system estrogen has its primary action on neural circuitry for lordosis. Finally, we have described how those neural circuitry changes foster behavioral changes that comprise increases in sexual motivation or "sex drive."

In summary, the interaction of estrogen with the neural circuitry for lordosis behavior as described in this book and briefly characterized above comprises an adequate neural mechanism for increased sexual motivation in female rats.

E.   Ethological Concepts: Their Physiological Realization

The neural circuitry for a natural mammalian behavior pattern and hormone effects upon it should have relevance for some of the concepts of ethology as formulated from the animal behavior studies of Lorenz (1950) and Tinbergen (1951). In fact, the neural and neuroendocrine mechanisms described for lordosis behavior can provide physiological explanations of phenomena that are essentially ethological. Neurobiological approaches to these behavioral issues are turning out to be exciting and successful (Huber, 1978). For a particular mammalian behavior response, we can try to match behavioral observations to some key ethological concepts to see if a physiological explanation has been approached.

The ethological concept of a *sign stimulus* is that a selected set of stimulus energies is required to evoke a selected behavioral response. A stimulus triggering a given behavioral response does not excite all receptors of all sense organs in the recipient animal (Tinbergen, 1951); instead, a "releasing mechanism," comprised essentially of a stimulus-filtering process, provides the key to the relevant motor mechanism. The essence of this concept is that it is a restricted set of stimuli that is relevant for triggering a given natural behavior. The facts surrounding lordosis behavior fit this concept perfectly. Stimuli for evoking lordosis behavior are restricted as to their modality. Only somatosensory information is necessary and sufficient for evoking lordosis in female rats. Among somatosensory stimuli, only cutaneous input from certain places on the skin of the female rat (ventral flank, posterior rump, and perineum) is relevant. Finally, even on those skin locations, stimuli involving cutaneous pressure are required. Thus, stimuli for lordosis behavior, whether provided by the male rat or by artificial cutaneous stimulation by the experimenter, fit the definition of sign stimuli. In turn, electrophysiological recording of the relevant input from primary sensory neurons and from interneurons in the spinal cord, along with circuitry analyses of how lordosis behavioral responses occur, provides a physiological explanation of how a sign stimulus works.

The concept of *fixed action pattern* is a natural behavioral response that is a movement of constant form. The definition includes the idea that subunits of the behavior, where recognized, have a fixed relation to each other. The basic description of lordosis behavior based on high-speed film and X-ray analyses (Chapter 1) and on anatomical and physiological studies of the muscular basis for response execution (Chapter 11) obviously fits the definition of a fixed action pattern. The mere achievement of a reliable description shows that the fixed action pattern concept is sufficient for characterizing lordosis behavior. In response to the sign stimulus, the vertebral dorsiflexion of lordosis always occurs in the female rat with adequate hormonal preparation. Within the vertebral dorsiflexion pattern, the subunit of greatest biological importance, elevation of the rump, is initiated first and is of most constant form. Thus, the explanation of the neural circuitry of and hormone action on lordosis behavior is an explanation of the physiological basis for a fixed action pattern.

Finally, Lorenz's "hydraulic" model of the motivation for instinctive behavioral responses can be used to describe the hormonal effects on rodent mating behavior. Operationally, from a "black box" point of view, estrogen provides the "pressure" for the lordosis behavior response to occur. Neurally, by its action on cells in and around the ventromedial nucleus of the hypothalamus, estrogen provides a behaviorally relevant increase in excitatory output to cells in and around the midbrain central gray. Over time, this prepares descending neurons in the lateral reticulospinal and lateral vestibulospinal systems such that when the sign stimulus enters at lumbar spinal cord levels, the vertebral dorsiflexion of lordosis behavior will occur. This increased descending excitation—from ventromedial hypothalamus, to midbrain central gray, to medullary reticulospinal system, to lumbar cord—provides a physiological realization of the "hydraulic" model of Lorenz.

Thus, the phenomena of female reproductive behavior in rodents are not only consistent with some of the key concepts of ethology; their neural and endocrine analysis also provides physiological explanations for ethological concepts in an interesting context.

F.   Progesterone Enhancement of Estrogen Action: Likely Mechanisms and Pathways Involved

Estrogen action on female reproductive behavior in rodents is enhanced by progesterone (Beach, 1948; Young, 1961). We have thoroughly examined mechanisms of estrogen action first because, in time of administration, it is the primary steroid hormone operating, and also because under some conditions it can act alone (without progesterone) on lordosis behavior (Davidson et al., 1968; Pfaff, 1970b). Furthermore, specific receptor mechanisms for estrogen, as revealed, for instance, by autoradiography (Chapter 6), make estrogen an attractive subject for primary study. Nevertheless, for a given dose of estrogen, higher levels of female rodent reproductive behavior can be obtained if estrogen action is facilitated by progesterone. Moreover, the time course of variations in lordosis behavior at the very beginning of estrogen administration and following temination of estrogen treatment parallel hypothalamic progesterone receptor levels (Madlafusek and Reynaud, 1979; Parsons, Mac-Cluskey, Pfaff, and McEwen, 1980). Therefore, it is useful to consider neural mechanisms and pathways involved in the mechanism of progesterone action (Kow, Malsbury and Pfaff, 1974b).

The theory of the neural mechanisms and pathways involved in progesterone facilitation of lordosis behavior, outlined in Figure 12–1, originated with previously published notions about the relationship between serotonin and female mating behavior in rodents. The anatomical relationships of serotonin neurons in the midbrain raphe nuclei became of special interest. Similarities between the effects of raphe lesions and septal lesions on several behavior patterns (Kow et al., 1974b) prompted us to formulate the hypothesis outlined below.

It appears that progesterone inhibits activity in a raphe–septal loop that includes serotonergic fibers and has the effect of inhibiting lordosis (Figure 12–1). Projections from the midbrain raphe nuclei through serotonergic fibers in the medial forebrain bundle or through fibers in the fasciculus retroflexus–stria medullaris system directly or indirectly reach the septum (Conrad, Leonard, and Pfaff, 1974). Projections from the septum through the medial forebrain bundle or through the stria medullaris–fasciculus retroflexus route directly or indirectly reach the midbrain raphe nuclei. Hypothalamic cells, including the progesterone-sensitive ones, can participate in this midbrain–limbic loop, at least through the medial forebrain bundle.

The dynamics of the raphe–septal loop normally maintain its neurons in a continually excitatory state. The net effect of descending brainstem projections from the loop is to inhibit responses to somatosensory input, thereby inhibiting lordosis. Interruption of function in the loop, by lesions or by antiserotonergic agents, facilitates responses to somatosensory input, thereby facilitating lordosis. Therefore, if progesterone decreases the activity or responses of neurons in this loop, it can facilitate lordosis (Figure 12–1). Data from the original experimental reports generating and supporting this model are given in the initial theoretical publication (Kow et al., 1974b).

The inhibitory effects of serotonin on lordosis behavior must be due to the ascending projections from midbrain raphe serotonergic nuclei, rather than the descending serotonergic projections from the medulla to the spinal cord. Indeed, serotonergic receptor stimulants acting in female rats with complete spinal transections (substituting for serotonergic endings of projections from medulla to spinal cord) actually increase the strength of some components of lordosis (Kow et al., 1980b). Therefore,

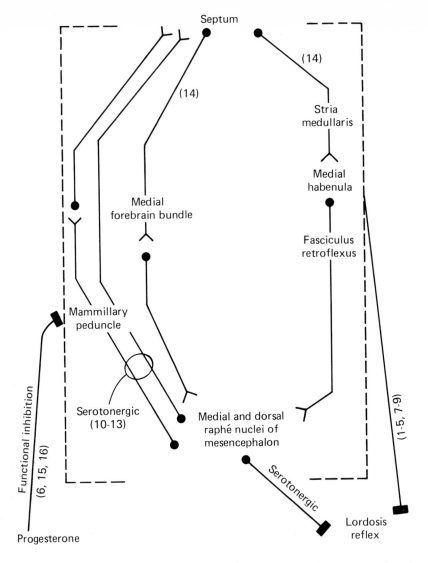

Figure 12–1. Model for the possible action of progesterone on lordosis in female rats. Progesterone is assumed to have a net inhibitory effect on a system of neurons linking the midbrain raphe nuclei with the septum. *Broken-line box:* these possibly progesterone-sensitive connections. *Lines on the left inside box:* projections through the medial forebrain bundle. Descending connections on reflex loops subserving lordosis could come via serotonergic fibers from the raphe nuclei themselves or from other parts of the raphe–septal system of connections. *Numbers in parentheses:* refer to correspondingly numbered paragraphs in the text of the original paper where the evidence is reviewed. —<, Excitatory relation; —■, inhibitory relation. (From Kow et al., 1974b)

the only major serotonergic cell groups remaining to serve the reproduction–inhibiting function described above are the midbrain raphe nuclei, as hypothesized above.

Progesterone effects mediated through effects on serotonin and raphe neurons may not have a great deal of behavioral specificity. Other behaviors may have the same relations as lordosis to the activity of medial hypothalamic, midbrain central gray, and raphe neurons. Schmitt, Paunovic, and Karli (1979) studied effects of raphe lesions on avoidance responses following medial hypothalamic stimulation. Midbrain central gray lesions caused a decline in the effect of ventromedial hypothalamic stimulation. In contrast, raphe lesions tended to enhance the ventromedial hypothalamic effect. Thus, this avoidance response has exactly the same relationship to hypothalamic, central gray, and raphe activity as lordosis behavior. This result emphasizes the potential multiple behavioral potency of some descending brainstem influences. In such a case, how may specific behavioral occurrences be explained in particular circumstances? This question is answered in the next section.

G. Economy in the Use of Descending Motor Executive Commands: The Issue of Behavioral Specificity

When a stimulus impinges on an organism, why does one behavioral response appear and not another? When descending commands in brainstem–spinal systems arrive at spinal cord segmental levels, why is one response facilitated and not another? These are questions of behavioral specificity.

The answer lies in the *codetermination* of any particular behavioral response by a specific stimulus input and a specific form of foregoing neural preparation. A stimulus impinging on a female rat will evoke lordosis behavior if and only if the neural tissue has been prepared by adequate steroid hormone action (registered in the cord through reticulospinal influences). Preparative aspects of estrogen and progesterone effects may well be heightened by foregoing chains of responses that, through behavioral dynamics, produce cascade effects (Section 2) and, through vestibular and neural dynamics, produce a state of great motor excitability (Section 3). Thus prepared, interneurons and motoneurons at lumbar cord levels allow lordosis behavior, but not other behaviors, to appear.

In regard to descending motor commands, selective requirements for subsequent stimulus input are the key to behavioral specificity. Given heightened activity in lateral reticulospinal and lateral vestibulospinal systems (exaggerated dramatically by positive feedback phenomena as explained in Sections 2 and 3), specific stimulus inputs can play upon lumbar interneurons and motoneurons as well-trained fingers can select a melody on a well-tuned piano. Lordosis behavior will appear if and only if the cutaneous pressure stimuli described in detail above actually occur.

1. Economical Use of Descending Axons for Controlling Motor Systems

The number of discrete responses by a mammalian organism, including all discriminable gradations of individual acts and all combinations of these acts, is extremely large. Considering this large number, it is obvious that it would be inefficient, if not impossible, to designate one or more axons in descending systems to be specifically devoted to each possible behavioral act. That type of descending system arrangement would have guaranteed behavioral specificity in descending motor commands; its absence means that the behavioral specificity we observe (for instance, in reproductive behavior phenomena) must be explained by other principles.

In fact, the specificity observed in the phenomena surrounding lordosis behavior can be explained by preparative actions of steroid hormones on the nervous system, spread over time, plus resultant positive feedback phenomena in the behavioral dynamics (Section 2) and neural dynamics (Section 3) of courtship behavior, plus the existence of specific stimulus requirements for lordosis described in Chapter 2. The effect of these sources of behavioral specificity is exactly to allow economy in the use of axons in descending motor control systems. With these sources of specificity, single axons "labeled" for individual behavioral acts are not needed.

The apparent absence of unnecessary specificity in the use of descending axons—that is, the selective designation of specific motor tasks by descending system axons only where and to the extent needed—corresponds to our "need to know" principle in the use of axons in ascending systems.

2. Chains of Response Can Produce a Cascade Effect

Selective stimulation at spinal cord levels as a key for explaining behavioral specificity actually can be divided into two parts according to the time of stimulus occurrence. The obvious part, referred to above, is the selective stimulation coming in from the skin (due either to the male rat or to artificial experimenter-generated input) at or just before the time of lordosis triggering. More subtle is the stimulus-responsive state produced by the female having gone through a chain of behavioral responses before the time at which the male rat contacts her skin. The behavioral dynamics in the chain of courtship responses aid behavioral specificity by producing a specific behavioral (and therefore neural) state in the female rat.

Under the influence of estrogen and progesterone, the courtship behavior of a female rat includes a hopping and darting form of loco-motion characterized by sudden movements forward with sudden stops. The sudden stops leave the female in a posture prepared to support the weight of the male during mounting (Figure 12–2; Pfaff et al., 1972). At this point the female is also in a muscularly tensed posture known to facilitate lordosis behavior; this state of muscular tension is probably due to the vestibular and neural dynamics recounted in Section 3. The "ear wiggling" (really head wiggling) of female rat courtship behavior facilitates the same state of muscular tension, probably also due to these vestibular and neural dynamics (Pfaff and Modianos, 1980). The produc-tion of this state in the female rat fosters behavioral specificity: it allows the subsequent triggering of lordosis behavior rather than another behav-ior upon contact from the male rat.

The effects of courtship behavior can also be routed through the male

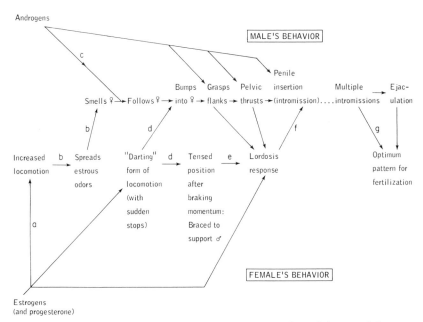

Figure 12–2. Flow chart of events in rat mating behavior, giving partial account of how endocrine secretions and behavioral determinants synchronize behavior of male and female to ensure reproduction. Time reads from left to right. Odor-spreading behavior of female (far left) may occur on the night before ovulation, while most of the events on the right occur on the night of ovulation. Small letters refer to notes and references in original paper. (From Pfaff et al., 1972)

rat in such a manner as to produce a cascade effect. The sudden stops in the hopping and darting form of locomotion encourage the male to bump into the female from the rear, in the correct position for mounting (Figure 12–2). Once cutaneous contact from the male begins, reproductive response components by the hormonally prepared female serve to facilitate subsequent stimulus application by the male, leading, again in a cascade manner, to the production of the full lordosis posture (Figure 1–5; Pfaff et al., 1972). Thus, courtship responses and initial lordosis components foster behavioral specificity in the sense that they encourage stimuli that lead to lordosis behavior (with the female in the appropriate hormonal state) and not other behaviors.

To put it another way, the behavioral encounter involves the androgen-prepared male in a state of sexual arousal and the estrogen–progesterone-prepared female. Their behavioral response chains are matched and synchronized in an adaptive fashion so as to produce a cascading sequence of responses leading to the full lordosis posture, intromission, and fertilization. The same behavioral cascade fosters behavioral specificity.

The production of the selective behavioral response in this way takes the load off the individual neurons in the motor and sensory pathways for lordosis behavior that act at the time of lordosis triggering. Less immediate specificity is required from their electrophysiological responses, because the state of the female (produced by the chain of courtship responses and initial lordosis components up to that time) has had its own selective effects. At time T, the female rat's specific response to the immediate stimulus is in part a result of that stimulus and in part a result of the behavioral and neural situation set up by preceding events. Thus, chains of responses producing cascades (sometimes routed through the stimulus-producing behavior of the male) place an upper limit on the requirements for immediate neuronal specificity in motor or sensory pathways, when explaining the selectivity of the behavioral outcome.

Similar principles apply to the female hamsters' reproductive behavior, which includes an elaborate signaling system. When not behaviorally receptive, female hamsters are very aggressive toward the male; the combined actions of estrogen and progesterone reduce this aggressiveness (Floody and Pfaff, 1974; Floody and Pfaff, 1977a,b). The female hamster uses olfactory signals and ultrasounds to communicate with the male (Figure 12–3; Floody and Pfaff, 1977a,b; Floody, Pfaff, and Lewis, 1977). She communicates to the male that under steroid hormone influence her aggressiveness is reduced and her sexual receptivity is increased, thus causing the male to approach (Figure 12–3). In turn, odors from the male foster female communicative behavior of this sort, and later lordotic behavior (Floody and Pfaff, 1977b; Floody et al., 1977; Noble, 1972, 1973). Thus, this chain of courtship responses by female hamsters (with causal effects that are routed through the male and

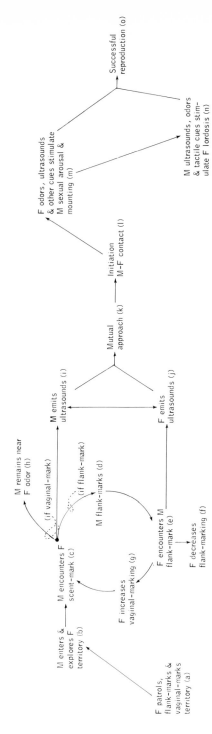

Figure 12–3. Summary of data describing a chain of social communications leading to reproduction in the golden hamster. Male behavior (*M*), above; female behavior (*F*), below. Lower case letters in parentheses code behavior elements for discussion in the text of the original paper. Many of the "links" in this chain of behaviors depend on gonadal hormones. In particular, testosterone facilitates male responses at least at points *d*, *h*, *m*, and *o*. Estrogen and progesterone facilitate female responses at least at points *a*, *g*, *j*, *k*, *n*, and *o*. (From Floody & Pfaff, 1977b)

involve a signaling system) also produces a behavioral state favorable for lordosis, intromission, and fertilization.

3. Chains of Courtship Responses Preparatory for Lordosis: Reflections on Neural State

The existence of courtship behaviors that occur well before lordosis and depend upon the actions of estrogen and progesterone is consistent with the notion of long-term preparative actions by these hormones. As recounted above, these courtship responses lead to states of excitation that foster lordosis. Thus, courtship responses in female rats are both a sign of a certain state of neural (and muscular) excitability and a cause of further elevation of this excitation. The neural dynamics by which this occurs are clarified in part below.

As described in Chapter 10, female rat courtship responses, including the sudden acceleration of hopping and darting and the rapid head movements involved in ear wiggling, reflect a high state of excitation in motor systems. In turn, stimulation of the vestibular organs due to these accelerations would cause an even higher pitch of excitation in the lateral vestibulospinal system. This causal sequence comprises a positive feedback system: from vestibulospinal excitation to the head and body musculature which produces the courtship response, to the vestibular stimulation produced by the courtship response, to further vestibulospinal excitation. Eventually, upon contact by the male rat, this excitation of descending neural pathways and axial muscular systems (which has been raised by the positive feedback loop) helps to guarantee that lordosis will occur.

In this context, the dependence of courtship responses in female rats on progesterone is especially interesting, and the mechanism of progesterone's action on lordosis (Section F) is further clarified. As specified in the model pictured in Figure 12-1, simply by inhibiting the repressive action of a serotonergic midbrain–limbic loop, progesterone can raise the level of active responses to somatosensory input. The overall increase in muscular responsivity thus produced raises the sensitivity of the somatosensory–vestibulospinal relationship to the operating range for the positive feedback system mentioned above to take over; that is, simple increases in the level of muscular excitability in response to somatosensory input essentially close the positive feedback loop, which allows the courtship behaviors to occur that produce the neural and behavioral cascade phenomena that foster the eventual lordosis reflex. Experiments testing the effects of progesterone in female rats not only on courtship behaviors but also on vestibulospinal and electromyographic measures will test this interpretation of the mechanisms involved. Interactions with the effects of serotonergic drugs are expected.

At the behavioral level, analogies between the cascade effects of courtship behavior in female rats and female hamsters are strong. However, hamsters mate in burrows, whereas rats mate in the open. Under these circumstances, it is not clear whether to expect the same dynamics of increased vestibulospinal and muscular excitability as a sign and cause of courtship behavior in female hamsters. Indeed, the decreased aggressiveness induced by progesterone in female hamsters might lead one to expect a different dynamic.

4. Summary: Behavioral States Fostering Behavioral Acts

Thus, an effect of response chains such as courtship behavior in female rats is to produce a neural *state* that fosters a subsequent behavioral *act*, i.e., lordosis. We can thus rely less on concurrent nerve cell responses for the explanation of the specificity of lordosis behavior: why lordosis and not another response occurs following adequate cutaneous input. From the point of view of the immediate cutaneous pressure stimulus, the lumbar spinal cord is prepared for the selection of lordosis. From the point of view of the hormone-dependent descending influence, the specific cutaneous pressure stimulus is also the key to selecting the reproductive behavior response.

In this way, the behavioral specificity lies in the recent "history" of the organism's behavior and relevant nerve cells. In rodent mating behavior, the chain of recent stimuli and responses produces a neural state (especially in the lateral vestibulospinal and reticulospinal systems) that determines the response potential of the animal. The controlling influences for this effect are found in the dynamics of the cascade and positive feedback systems described above. Behaviorally, the foregoing courtship responses and early copulatory responses by the female allow subsequent stimulus presentation by the male, leading, in loop form, to further responses by the female. Neurally, excitation in the vestibulospinal–musculature–vestibular–vestibulospinal system is raised in the manner of a positive feedback loop.

The very existence of courtship responses that depend on estrogen and progesterone is evidence that hormone-dependent influences descending from the brainstem to the spinal cord can prepare the way for the eventual lordosis response; that is, important aspects of steroid hormone action have a preparative, as opposed to reflexive, neural and behavioral role (Figure 12–4). Estrogen and progesterone are not limited to enhancing stimulus–brainstem–spinal cord reflexes by virtue of their effects on brainstem and hypothalamic nerve cell responses to current sensory input; rather, they can have actions which, over a period of time, prepare lower brainstem and spinal cord neurons for behavior triggering that can be essentially spinal. This effect is consistent with the slow time course of estrogen action on nerve cells (Chapter 6; Parsons, Krieger, McEwen, and Pfaff, 1980). It is also consistent with an absence

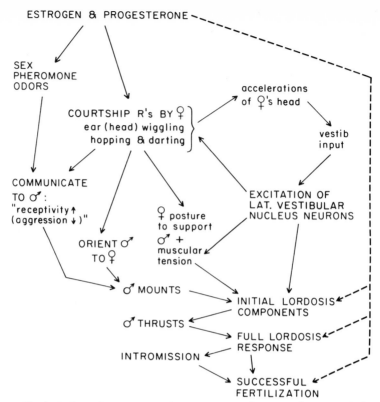

Figure 12–4. Roles of estrogen and progesterone in preparing neural circuitry so that lordosis behavior can occur. Such preparation can include the prior display of courtship (proceptive) behaviors by the female.

of convincing responses by midbrain central gray neurons that project to the medullary reticular formation (Sakuma and Pfaff, 1980b) and the lack of responses to lordosis-relevant stimulation in medullary reticulospinal neurons recorded in unanesthetized preparations (Kow and Pfaff, 1980).

The time course of preparation by nerve cells for the occurrence of lordosis may reflect how far anterior in the neuraxis those nerve cells are located. Obviously, interneurons at lumbar levels of the spinal cord would have to be prepared to receive relevant, current sensory input; but even there, the relatively weak monosynaptic reflex of relevant epaxial motoneurons allows for strong previous descending facilitation (Chapter 11). In the medulla, reticulospinal neurons and lateral vestibulospinal neurons integrate slower postural changes covering the entire vertebral axis. The time course of the recovery of lordosis behavior following subtotal nucleus gigantocellularis lesions parallels that of the recovery of axial posture independent of locomotion (Zemlan et al., 1980a). Likewise, in female rats with massive destruction of the cerebellum, we found that if the animal could stand, she could perform lordosis irrespective of whether or not she could walk (Zemlan and Pfaff, 1975). The changes originating with hypothalamic neurons appeared to be even slower. The electrophysiological nature of these cells (Chapter 6) and, especially, the effects of estrogen on these cells appear to be related to the slow rhythms of the endocrine system rather than the millisecond-by-millisecond time course of conventional nerve cell action. Nevertheless, estrogen action on these cells in the hypothalamus is effective in facilitating reproductive behavior. Therefore, there must be a tonic mode of action (as opposed to reflexive): estrogen must have the role, mediated by hypothalamic cells, of preparing lower brainstem neurons and, in turn, lumbar spinal cord interneurons.

H.   Achieving Unity in an Organism's Action

Endocrine and behavioral actions of an organism must be appropriate to the environment in which they occur (Table 12–1). According to the length of gestation, increasing day length and environmental temperature help to ensure that the young will be born at a time of year such that environmental conditions will favor their survival. Reproduction is unlikely without an adequate food supply. Absence of stress (e.g., relative safety from predators, absence of signals from conspecifics due to crowding, or other factors) may be required.

Table 12-1. Endocrine and behavioral preparations for reproduction

Need for coordination	Tissue	Substance
Appropriate endocrine & behavioral responses to environment	sensory systems & central neural inputs to hypothalamus	—
Synchrony of endocrine preparation for reproduction with behavioral	Hypothalamic nerve cells	
	Input	Steroid hormones (estrogen + progesterone)
	Output	Peptide hormone LHRH
Behavioral synchrony of ♀ with ♂	Courtship & lordosis neural circuitry	—
Endocrine synchrony of ovulation with uterine preparation	Ovary	Steroid hormones (estrogen + progesterone)

Given that reproduction is to occur, endocrine preparations must be synchronized with behavior. Ovulation in the female and spermatogenesis in the male must begin at such a time that when copulation occurs fertilization is possible. On the behavioral side, male and female must find and approach each other and copulate. They are brought together by courtship signals and copulatory sequences that comprise a behavioral funnel. After the sperm and egg have joined, the genital tract of the female must be ready for implantation.

How are these requirements for integration met? The mechanism involves at least five types of tissue in the female: sense organs, central nervous system including hypothalamus, pituitary, ovary, and uterus. It employs at least four types of chemical messages between cells: neurotransmitters, peptide-releasing hormones, protein hormones (LH and FSH), and steroid hormones. A model of the influences governing reproductive behavior shows how this integration occurs (Figure 12–5).

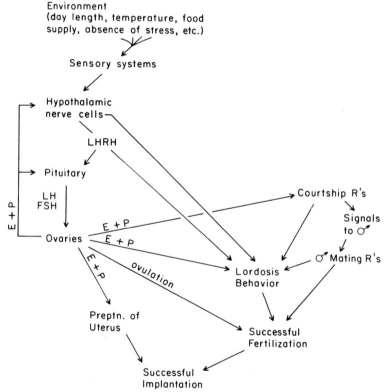

Figure 12–5. Roles of neural and endocrine tissues, using peptide and steroid hormones, in integrating an organisms's behavioral and endocrine responses with its environment to foster successful reproduction. *E*, estrogen; *P*, progesterone; *R's*, responses; *LHRH*, luteinizing hormone releasing hormone; *LH*, luteinizing hormone; *FSH*, follicle stimulating hormone.

1. Hypothalamic Nerve Cells Adapt Endocrine, Behavioral, and Autonomic Responses to Environmental Constraints

Hypothalamic nerve cells receive information about day length (at least) through the suprachiasmatic nuclei. They are sensitive to changes in body temperature (at least) through specialized thermoreceptors in the preoptic area. Information about food supply is required, in any case, for the direction of feeding behavior by cells in the ventromedial nucleus of the hypothalamus. Information about stress, for instance in the form of somatosensory input due to pain or the contact resulting from crowding, comes over ascending pathways from the mesencephalic central gray. Thus, hypothalamic nerve cells receive inputs that are suited to the regulation of reproduction according to important environmental variables.

Hypothalamic outputs governing reproduction according to environmental constraints are both behavioral and endocrine. The endocrine outputs are the releasing hormones that influence pituitary protein hormone release. The primary behavioral output in the female rodent is lordosis behavior; the hypothalamic mechanisms governing this behavior were set forth in Chapter 7. In turn, for the synchrony required between female and male behaviors, courtship signals operate as described in Chapter 12, Section G. Finally, autonomic changes consistent with the required skeletal behavioral acts are controlled by hypothalamic nerve cells as reviewed in Chapter 7, Section C and illustrated in Figure 7–10.

2. Peptide-Releasing Hormones Synchronize Behavioral with Endocrine Events

Dramatically, lordosis behavior in the female rat is coordinated in part with ovulation through the action of a single substance, luteinizing hormone-releasing hormone LHRH. Working through the portal circulation, LHRH leads to the release of LH from the pituitary, which causes ovulation. LHRH also has effects on other nerve cells that promote female reproductive behavior, leading to fertilization (Moss and McCann, 1973, 1975; Pfaff, 1973). In fact, an antibody against LHRH applied to nerve cells in the central gray, in the region of hypothalamic axon termination, can block lordosis behavior (Sakuma and Pfaff, 1980a). The integration by LHRH means that ovulation will occur at about the same time as the sperm is allowed (behaviorally) to enter the genital tract, thus fostering fertilization.

In this context, protein hormones such as LH and FSH simply carry the message (from the pituitary to the ovaries) to stimulate ovarian hormone production (estrogen and progesterone) and gametogenesis (leading to ovulation) at an appropriate time.

3. Steroid Hormones Synchronize Behavioral Acts, Ovulation, and Uterine Preparation

As seen in Figure 12–5, the steroid hormones estrogen (*E*) and progesterone (*P*) play a central role in coordinating preparation for reproduction by the brain, pituitary, ovary, and uterus. On a broad time scale, the same ovarian activation responsible for gametogenesis, leading to ovulation, accounts for steroidogenesis, leading to the production of estrogen and progesterone, which will cause the hormonal stimulation of the genital tract. At the same time, these steroid hormones have feedback actions on the brain and pituitary which regulate pituitary protein hormone release. Finally, the actions of estrogen and progesterone on female reproductive behavior have been documented in Chapters 1, 2, and 6.

4. Can We Generalize?

Our model of the female rodent's preparations for reproduction may provide a paradigm for showing how behavioral responses controlled by neural circuitry (and hormone action) can be orchestrated to induce actions consistent with environmental constraints on the one hand and internal physiological requirements on the other. All the environmental signals to be considered must be brought together in one place. For the control of reproduction, that place is a set of nerve cells in the preoptic area and hypothalamus. It is possible to unify outputs by means of the various actions of a single substance. In reproductive physiology this substance is LHRH. However, it is not necessary to have a single substance to achieve integration, and LHRH is probably not the only means by which endocrine–behavioral integration is achieved in the hypothalamic mechanisms for reproduction. LHRH has a limited distribution of targets; it travels through the portal circulation to act on the pituitary and a limited number of other nerve cells. The integrative power of other substances derives precisely from their wide distribution. Through the general circulation steroid hormones reach, and therefore can synchronize activities in, brain tissue, the pituitary, and the uterus (Figure 12–5).

Finally, within an organ, functions can be linked to achieve important integrative effects. In the ovary, coordination of gametogenesis leading to ovulation with the production of estrogen has this effect (Figure 12–5).

Chapter 13
Summary

We can follow the flow of action potentials through the neural pathways for lordosis, from the application of stimuli by the male to the initiation of lordosis behavior by the female. This comprises the simplest possible neural mechanism for this mammalian reproductive behavior.

During the natural course of mating behavior in rats, the male grasps the flanks of the female and thrusts against her posterior rump, tailbase, and perineum. Cutaneous stimulation of her flanks, followed by pressure on her posterior rump, tailbase, and perineum skin are necessary and sufficient for lordosis.

These stimuli cause a barrage of action potentials from most of the cutaneous responsive unit types in the relevant dorsal root ganglia; for example, perineal stimuli excite neurons in dorsal root ganglion L_6. However, among all the types of primary sensory neurons, only pressure units and Type I units give sustained responses to the cutaneous pressure required for lordosis. The stimulus requirements for the pressure units to fire most closely fit those for the lordosis behavior response. Summation across pressure units must occur for lordosis to be initiated. Thus, if any single chain of sensory events has the central role, it is the following: pressure on the crucial skin areas deforms Ruffini endings, activating pressure-sensitive primary neurons (Figure 13–1).

Input from primary sensory units responsive to pressure converges on pressure-sensitive interneurons in the intermediate gray of the lumbar spinal cord of female rats. Stimulus activation of these interneurons at spinal cord segmental levels is the main way in which adequate stimulation triggers lordosis behavior. Convergence on interneurons forms the mechanism by which stimulus summation can drive the behavior.

Since female rats with the spinal cord isolated from higher neural centers do not perform lordosis, some type of supraspinal facilitation must be required. Insofar as ascending fibers participate, those which could be relevant for lordosis behavior terminate in the medullary

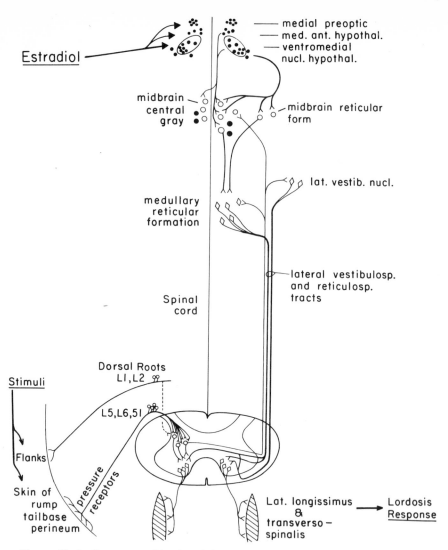

Figure 13–1. Summary of basic minimal neural circuitry for lordosis behavior, from stimulus to response, and including estrogen effect. Component neural systems are summarized in greater detail, where knowledge allows, in the summary figures of previous chapters. In this behavior, stimuli, responses, circuitry, and hormone effects are all bilateral, and are shown here on just one side for convenience.

reticular formation, in the lateral vestibular nucleus, and in and around the midbrain central gray. However, the frequency of occurrence and nature of responses to cutaneous stimulation by nerve cells in these brainstem target areas suggest that they do not control lordosis simply by responding strongly and promptly to stimulation on lordosis-relevant skin areas. In addition to any role these brainstem neurons have in spinal–brainstem–spinal reflex action, they also must facilitate lordosis over a longer period of time, in a tonic fashion. This action, in part, reflects the time course of the estrogen influences that originate in the hypothalamus.

The distribution of sensory information to brainstem neurons participating in lordosis control is spare and is not very precise in space or time. It does not need to be. Thus, the modest role of lordosis-relevant stimulus information ascending to the brainstem reflects economy in the use of neural signaling capacity. In turn, lordosis-relevant neurons in the midbrain central gray and medullary reticular formation facilitate the behavioral response primarily by carrying descending hormone-dependent influences initiated in the medial hypothalamus.

Decerebrate female rats, with complete disconnection of the diencephalon and forebrain from the lower brainstem and spinal cord, do not perform lordosis. Therefore, certain cells in the diencephalon or forebrain must provide an obligatory facilitatory influence. Among them, only cells in and around the ventromedial nucleus of the hypothalamus qualify as the source of the behavior-facilitating descending signal. Lesions of these cells lead to lordosis loss. Electrical stimulation of these cells at low frequencies facilitates lordosis behavior. Cells in the medial hypothalamus may facilitate the lordosis response in part by elevating luteinizing hormone releasing hormone (LHRH) release onto other neurons. This would provide a mechanism with a suitably slow time course of action on midbrain cells. In any case, a sure means by which ventromedial hypothalamic cells control lordosis is through the local facilitating effects of estrogen on these cells.

Estrogen is required for lordosis to occur. To facilitate the behavior, estrogen blood levels must have been raised for at least 20 hours. The hormone can act to promote lordosis by local effects on cells in and lateral to the ventromedial nucleus of the hypothalamus.

In all vertebrate species, cells in specific groups in the medial hypothalamus (as well as in the medial preoptic area and certain limbic forebrain structures) accumulate estrogen. For each species the locations of estrogen- or androgen-binding cells can be correlated with the control of hormone-dependent pituitary or behavioral functions. In the brain of the female rat, cells in the ventromedial nucleus of the hypothalamus, especially in its ventrolateral subdivision and just ventral and lateral to it, strongly concentrate radioactive estrogen. Estrogen can increase the electrical activity of slowly firing cells in this region and can increase the ultrastructural signs of biosynthetic activity. Through these cellular effects, estrogen can cause a tonically elevated output from the ventromedial hypothalamus to the midbrain, which facilitates lordosis.

Medial hypothalamic cells integrate behavioral responses with other aspects of the physiology of the organism. The nature of their control of both female and male reproductive behavior coordinates behavioral mechanisms with autonomic controls. Steroid hormone effects on hypothalamic cells, as well as hypothalamic influences on pituitary hormone release, coordinate endocrine function with behavior.

Progesterone facilitates estrogen actions on lordosis behavior. Its behavioral effect appears to be related to activity in a midbrain–limbic loop which includes serotonergic cells, and which inhibits responses to somatosensory input, including lordosis. By decreasing activity in this loop, progesterone facilitates lordosis.

Axons descending from the medial hypothalamus and preoptic area to the midbrain do so with a degree of anatomical order: those exiting from more medially placed cell bodies tend to have stronger medial running trajectories; those exiting from more laterally placed cell bodies tend to have stronger lateral trajectories; and those exiting from more dorsally placed cell bodies tend to have stronger dorsal trajectories. Axons descending in sheets from more anteriorly placed groups of cell bodies in the basal forebrain tend to run in sheets wrapped, laterally, around those from more posteriorly placed cell body groups as they descend toward the midbrain, in a manner reminiscent of laminar flow.

The hypothalamic axons most important for lordosis control, those descending from the ventromedial nucleus, run toward the midbrain in two groups. One group of axons circles far laterally and then descends to the midbrain, while the other goes straight back through the medial hypothalamus, reaching the midbrain through the periventricular system.

The medial- and lateral-running groups of ventromedial hypothalamic axons descending to the midbrain comprise an asymmetrical OR gate with respect to lordosis control. Either can substitute to some extent for the other, but quantitatively the lateral-running fibers make the more important contribution. They both act through their connections in the midbrain, in or near the central gray. Electrical stimulation in the midbrain central gray can facilitate lordosis. Central gray lesions disrupt it.

The activity of central gray neurons reflects hypothalamic and hormonal influences. Factors that increase lordosis behavior (estrogen and electrical stimulation of the ventromedial hypothalamus) raise the excitability of certain central gray nerve cells. Factors that decrease lordosis (such as input from the medial preoptic area) can lower central gray nerve cell excitability.

Some cells in the midbrain central gray send out axons that descend to the reticular formation of the lower brainstem, including the ventral portion of the medullary reticular formation. Midbrain signals important for lordosis control can be integrated and relayed to the spinal cord through contacts with reticulospinal cells in this region. From ventromedial hypothalamus to lumbar spinal cord, transfers from neuron to neuron preserve the relationship that increased cellular activity leads to increased lordosis.

Brainstem neurons that project to the spinal cord form a neural funnel through which hormonal influences (including those of estrogen, progesterone, and LHRH) must pass in order to influence reproductive behavior. The lateral vestibulospinal tract, descending from the lateral vestibular nucleus, and the lateral reticulospinal tract, descending from the nucleus gigantocellularis in the ventromedial medullary reticular formation, are the pathways that facilitate lordosis. Lesions of these descending systems lead to lordosis loss, whereas electrical stimulation of the lateral vestibular nucleus facilitates the behavior. These two descending pathways control motoneurons for axial muscles. They branch at different vertebral levels and act bilaterally. All of these properties are well suited to their roles in lordosis behavior.

The lateral reticulospinal and lateral vestibulospinal tracts help in part to prepare lumbar spinal circuits for the initiation of lordosis. With input from the midbrain central gray, reticulospinal cells can relay estrogen-dependent hypothalamic signals, transmitted via the midbrain, to the spinal cord. The lateral vestibulospinal nucleus lacks such direct input from the hypothalamus or midbrain central gray. It elevates the postural tone of axial muscles. In doing so it is susceptible to the facilitating influences of courtship behavior. Thus, working in concert, these two systems prepare lumbar circuits in such a manner as to facilitate reflex vertebral dorsiflexion. From their positions in the lower brainstem they can integrate postural adaptations across segmental levels over the length of the entire body axis. The specificity of their action in facilitating lordosis depends on the combination of their descending influences with the specific patterns of cutaneous pressure required for this behavior.

Branches of axons descending in the lateral reticulospinal and lateral vestibulospinal tracts allow axial motoneurons at various levels and on both sides of the spinal cord to receive descending excitatory influences. In female rats, the net result of their combined actions increases electrical excitability in motoneurons required for the reflex vertebral dorsiflexion of lordosis behavior. Indeed, the monosynaptic reflex for these axial motoneurons is weaker than expected (for example, from limb muscle motoneurons), allowing for a powerful effect of descending influences. The motoneurons involved represent the intersection of adequate sensory input at lumbar levels with adequate descending influences. They control the epaxial lateral longissimus and transversospinalis muscles, and their cell bodies lie on the medial and ventromedial borders of the ventral horn. They are located in spinal levels receiving dorsal roots from T_{12} through S_1.

The deep back muscles, the lateral longissimus and transversospinalis, execute the vertebral dorsiflexion of lordosis. They are anatomically connected so as to be competent to achieve dorsiflexion, and their electrical stimulation produces dorsiflexion. Their ablation reduces lordosis strength. Thus, these muscles are responsible for the rump elevation of lordosis—biologically, the most crucial component. The activation of the motoneurons controlling these muscles, by the combination of adequate sensory and sufficient descending influences, represents the end point of the neural and neuroendocrine control systems for lordosis. The occurrence of this mammalian reproductive behavior allows fertilization and subsequent impregnation.

Chapter 14
Epilogue

A. Computability: Can This Be Done?

It is not obvious whether or not one can achieve a complete and precise description of the neural mechanism for a behavior pattern in a mammalian brain. On the face of it, the large number of possible stimuli, the variety of possible responses, especially considering all gradations, and the extremely large number of combinations of stimuli and responses make the difficulties clear. At the neural level, the large number of nerve cells and the complexities of their connections are further evidence of the difficulty of this task.

As a problem, is the circuit for a mammalian behavior "solvable" in a finite time? In mathematics, some problems can be proven to be so difficult that their solution would require infinitely large computers or an infinite amount of time (Stockmeyer and Chandra, 1979). To prove a problem in neural analysis solvable, one must supply a precise description of the neural elements involved and a set of rules for the interactions among those elements such that, for any set of stimuli applied to the system, it can be decided by the application of these rules whether any given response will occur. Even though this is hard and has not formally been proven to be possible, it would also be tricky to prove that it is impossible. With the state of knowledge at any given time, a theorist trying to prove the task impossible would be hard pressed to guarantee that greater knowledge of nerve cells, better understanding of their interactions, and more efficient descriptions of their systematic behavior might not render the precise description of a behavioral mechanism achievable.

At this point we cannot prove the task mathematically possible; neither can we prove it impossible. Therefore, the only course of action is to continue empirical progress toward the actual description of the neural circuit for a mammalian behavior. Success in achieving this will have to be its own existence proof. The degree of completeness of our current understanding of the circuitry for lordosis is very encouraging.

In mathematical problems of extreme difficulty, the time required for solution rises exponentially as a function of the number of elements in the problem. One way in which the mathematical theorist can circumvent the dilemma of abstract unsolvability is to keep his problem manageably small. Clearly, this points the way to a useful strategy for the mammalian neurobiologist. Our first systematic attempts at a physiological explanation must focus on behavioral circumstances of relative simplicity in their stimulus and response content in order to avoid certain mathematical problems that occur when "all possible combinations" of stimulus and response contingencies are considered. Another way the mathematical theorist approaches abstract problems of unsolvability is to drop the requirement that he solve all instances of a given class of problems; he settles for a finite number of them. Likewise, the mammalian neurophysiologist must find a number of fortunate cases that have proven to be susceptible to behavioral and neural analysis. These must be simple enough to allow physiological experimentation, but complex enough to fit recognizably into adaptive behavior patterns. As in every other branch of science, principles of neural circuitry and operation generated from the exhaustive study of these particular systems would have then to be applied to all other cases.

1.   What Matters is What Counts—Or Is the Nervous System Logical?

If we are to achieve a precise description of a neural mechanism for a behavioral response, we need to use a formal language that is adequate. How shall the elements and interactions between elements be expressed such that rules and principles can be stated clearly? For many mathematicians, the usual approach to this type of biological problem would be to focus exclusively on numbers. Extrapolating from the legitimate experimental strategy of striving for quantification in neurobiology, some theorists might take the overly restrictive attitude that if a model does not exclusively use numbers, it doesn't count. The trouble with this approach is that it prematurely predisposes us to certain forms of mathematical expression, for example, calculus.

It is not yet obvious which formal language will be optimal for expressing the questions and solutions in neurobiology. For the description of the systematic behavior of neural networks which yield orderly behavioral responses, forms of symbolic logic should be considered. The similarity between the elements of threshold logic and some aspects of the operation of nerve cells has been encouraging. In Chapter 12, examples of how networks of threshold logic could be applied, for instance, to questions of neural convergence were considered. With the potential of handling large numbers of weighted inputs, whose sum at any given time might or might not reach threshold (which, itself, could be modulated), threshold elements produce strings of binary outputs (Dertouzos, 1965; Hill and Peterson, 1974; Kohavi, 1978). By using to advantage the theorems that have been developed for arrangement of these threshold logic elements, one might successfully model a neural circuit with as much known about it as, for instance, the circuit for lordosis behavior.

In turn, if we can express precisely the regularities of the circuitry and operations of the neural mechanism for a behavioral response such that it can be modeled on a computer (an easy step if threshold logic is used), we can prove in a formal sense that the problem is solvable. Turing, a British mathematician, proved that any precisely stated solution to a mathematical problem can be executed by a machine which is the equivalent of a simple computer. The demonstration that a mathematical problem can be solved by a "Turing machine," a simple computer, is a necessary and sufficient condition for saying that a problem is solvable by a complete and precise mathematical procedure (Stockmeyer and Chandra, 1979).

How do we decide which type of formal expression is most appropriate for a given neural system? Two approaches must be followed in parallel. First, continued experimentation to generate new information in well-studied neural–behavioral systems will make increasingly clear which forms of expression are best. Second, parallel attempts at modeling, using languages that appear to be reasonable first choices, will tell us which types of experimental information are needed to produce complete mechanistic answers within the scope of those models.

B.   Morality: Should This Be Done?

Should complete and precise descriptions of neural mechanisms for mammalian behavior patterns be attempted? Some philosophically in-clined writers have exhibited a mistrust of the behavioral and neural sciences in this regard. For example, William Irwin Thompson (1973) sometimes tries to belittle our efforts in a somewhat hysterical tone:

> In our physical sciences we have long since gone beyond the Eighteenth Century notion of dead hunks of matter moving in the black void of space. Yet our psychological sciences are still restricted to Eighteenth Century mechanistic notions: minds are simply located hunks of gray matter moving in the black void of time. (Thompson, 1973, p. 124)

At other points, Thompson seems to fear the power of the behavioral sciences:

> Had the materialists at home convinced us that the money for manned spaceflights should be spent on more pressing problems, they would also have convinced us that it should go to the experts in the field of behavioral problems, and a psychological inner space program would have arisen under the direction of men like Harvard's behavioral psychologist B. F. Skinner or Yale's psychosurgeon Jose M. Delgado. Under the misguided notion that we had to use our technology to solve our problems here on earth. . . . ''
> (Thompson, 1973, p. 6)

Thompson's attitudes seem arrogant and vaguely antiintellectual in that they caricature entire fields of honest scientific endeavor. They seem to be telling us that we should not use our intelligence to better our lot.

A more serious statement of the problem of control of neural and behavioral technology following scientific advances comes from the writing of B. F. Skinner (1953). In his view, physiological explanations of behavior have the same status as any other systematically expressed knowledge of behavioral causes. The problem is that the more detailed our understanding of the structure and mechanisms of human behavior, the more powerful the potential controls deriving from behavioral and neural technology can be.

Unfortunately, the potential behavioral controls generated by modern behavioral and neural methods may be used not only for purposes commonly agreed to be good, but also for controversial or clearly evil purposes.

To approach this problem, let us assume that human behavior is already, and will continue to be, under effective social control. If so, would it be smart, or even moral, to fail to use intelligent scientific means to understand how those controls operate? Our refusal to use the neural and behavioral sciences to understand behavioral mechanisms would not leave human behavior in a state of freedom, but would simply prolong our ignorance of the controls already limiting us. In addition to our genetic heritage, we are subjected to familial, religious, social, educational, and governmental limitations on our behavior. Under these conditions Skinner (1953) would say that blindly calling our behavior "free" would just be an excuse for leaving its causes unspecified.

Some may say, "better the existing controls than modified ones based on behavioral or neural sciences." How can a person argue against a better understanding of how existing controls work? Advanced behavioral and neural scientific knowledge would allow us to evaluate better the worth of existing controls and/or allow us to make them work better. In the last analysis, specifying the biological bases of behavior will permit us to understand the organism which understands, and to evaluate the organism which evaluates.

Thus, we need not focus exclusively on the negative side of the achievements of the behavioral and neural sciences; we can also look at the obvious positive benefits of the technology deriving from these fields. If they are worth the risk, the next step must be to guarantee adequate social regulation of the applications of behavioral and neural technology. Part of this task obviously must be to diversify decision-making power and to spread the control of behavioral technology among institutions and agencies, so that no one (potentially evil) group can gain inordinate control (Skinner, 1953). In fact, by the normal, wide distribution of scientific knowledge, especially via modern electronic media, we hope to ensure that the regulation of resulting technology cannot rest with a dangerously small number of individuals. Failure to opt for the orderly growth of the behavioral and neural sciences (and its potential benefits) will simply leave future nascent scientific advances in the hands of possibly immoral groups of individuals with less good will than ourselves.

The mechanistic approach to the biological explanation of behavior through physiology is only one approach that may be used; another is to show the partial determination of animal and human behavior by evolutionary constraints (E. O. Wilson, 1975, 1979). In recent years, sociobiology has coalesced creatively to summarize systematic studies of the social behavior of animals, especially as they reflect evolutionary processes. It also offers the possibility of understanding the biological adaptiveness of our human codes of ethics. To the extent that we neglect this opportunity, we are leaving the future of our ethical development to chance.

A source of mistrust and misunderstanding of neurobiological explanations of behavior has been the occasional view that systematic scientific approaches to behavior come from bad habits of Western thought (Bateson, 1979). According to this view the analysis of complex behavioral phenomena into smaller and simpler parts and the reduction of behavioral facts to explanations in terms of physiological variables will fail because complex phenomena uniquely require explanation at their own level. Antireductionist biases of this sort are also antiintellectual and obscurantist. We cannot prove ahead of time that neurobiology will explain behavior, but the intellectually straightforward approach is to try to do it systematically and, following achievement of a set of principles, to see what is left to be explained. The success of scientific explanation will have to be its own existence proof.

In summary, we must not only ask whether it is moral to pursue precise explanations of behavior, but also whether it is moral not to. We should use our most sophisticated, systematic, and intellectually powerful approaches to better our lot. In their most extended form neurobiological explanations of the mechanisms and adaptiveness of behavior should allow us to understand our system of values. Approaches to human morality are not fixed. During the Renaissance, antiquated forms of Christian ethics were transformed into a lay morality. Now, during the late twentieth and early twenty-first century, neurobiological insights into the emotions and motivations of animals and humans may further the development of a biologically based morality.

C.   Extrapolation to Human Affairs

How likely is it that forms of neural control over behavior discovered in experimental animals also operate in the human? Very likely, based on both general grounds and specific examples.

In general, during vertebrate evolution, neuroanatomy has been conservative. Passage from smaller to bigger brains has been accomplished not by losing tracts, but by adding them. The older ones are still there. For these tracts, given similar anatomical arrangements of cells and no indication that cells operate differently, we generally expect similar principles of neural control in humans as in experimental animals.

Many behaviors in humans remain analogous to animal behavior. Humans are required by the physical world not only to maintain posture against the force of gravity, but also to engage in certain regulatory behavior patterns. Internally, humans must respire, circulate blood, maintain blood pressure and body temperature, etc. In regard to the external world, they must secure food, water, safe habitat, mating partners, etc. Under these circumstances, we expect not only similar motivational patterns, but also emotional dispositions required for the attainment of these commodities.

More specifically, we found (Chapter 6) patterns of steroid hormone binding in brain true for every form of vertebrate we studied. Estrogens and androgens seem to be accumulated by certain medial hypothalamic and limbic nerve cells in every animal "from fish to philosopher." The same steroid hormones are produced and circulate in humans as in the experimental animals we studied. The principles of neuroendocrine feedback and phenomena such as ovulation do not seem to be different. Therefore, we expect similar endocrine–neural relationships in humans and in experimental animals.

Another, more startling example concerns a practical effect of steroid hormones. Many women have stopped using contraceptive pills because of their side effects on mood, mainly depression. In 1959, Kawakami and Sawyer published results of an electrophysiological study in rabbits showing progesterone effects on electroencephalographic patterns of arousal which signify a clear depressive effect of the hormone. In this case, electrophysiological results from an experimental animal could have been used to predict side effects of a birth control agent in humans.

In summary, when we compare experimental animals and humans, neuroanatomical patterns are conservative, endocrine principles are similar, and certain features of behavior remain the same. Therefore, we expect principles of the neural control of behavior to remain similar. Indeed, one task of this branch of medical science is to understand the human brain, which appreciates the human life that other branches of medical science attempt to prolong.

D.   Some Outstanding Questions

Although a summary of knowledge or a scientific theory is made as complete as possible at any given time, part of its usefulness is to provide a solid platform for new experiments. In this area of study, the most obvious step would be more detailed studies of cellular mechanisms through the application of modern cell biological techniques. The application of intracellular electrical recording techniques will allow us to study the convergence of influences on nerve cells known to be critical for behavior, where those convergences are revealed only in postsynaptic potentials. Electrical recording from cells in tissue slices will allow us to change the composition of the medium surrounding the cells in a manner impossible in vivo.

Further electron microscopic study of hormone-sensitive neurons and their endings should yield morphological results that will correlate with the known physiology of the cells and predict neurochemical events. One question is whether there are any morphological peculiarities of hormone-sensitive neurons which would allow their identification as such and which would give clues to their special role. Beyond that, the obvious questions concern the morphological nature of hormone effects on these cells.

The better the anatomical and physiological characterization of a behavioral mechanism and hormone effect, the more rational will be the chemical investigation of the nerve cells involved. One exciting line of neurochemical research connected with the work described in this book is the continuing study of cellular mechanisms of estrogen and progesterone action. Do relatively fast hormone effects, perhaps involving only cell membrane or cytoplasm, have any physiological role in estrogen action on nerve cells, or are cell nuclear alterations always required? Where estrogen causes changes in genomic readout, resulting in biosynthetic alterations, what is the nature of the new RNA and proteins synthesized?

Computer modeling of the neural circuitry for a behavioral response will be able to ensure precise and quantitative statements of our hypotheses about how the behavioral mechanism works, how steroid hormones affect it, and, therefore, how a motivational change occurs. In turn, formal statements of this sort allow objective criticism. Threshold logic provides one formal language for this modeling, but other logical and mathematical approaches may be better.

One direction for new research is thus toward the more detailed study of the cellular mechanisms for a behavioral response; another direction is toward a wider biologically integrative view. For example, the manner in which an individual behavioral response follows from the flow of behavior preceding it and sets up behaviors which will follow it has been a fascinating question since the time of Sherrington. More generally, an understanding of the biologically adaptive benefits of the ways in which certain behavioral responses are coordinated with endocrine and other organismic states and the ways in which those relationships in turn are made appropriate to the environment is fair game for new work. The precise delineation of the neural mechanism for a centrally placed behavioral response can be very helpful in thinking about these wider questions. Computer modeling will permit the rigorous statement of more integrative ideas of this sort. Attempts at making such statements will point the way toward the type of data needed for the adequate generation and testing of new ideas.

References

Abzug, C., Maeda, M., Peterson, B. W., and Wilson, V. J. (1974) Cervical branching of lumbar vestibulospinal axons. *J. Physiol., 243:* 499–522.

Ahmed, S. M. (1974) Electrocardiographic changes on hypothalamic stimulation in dog. XXVI International Congress of Physiological Sciences, New Delhi, Abstract 597, p. 199.

Alcaraz, M., Guzman-Flores, C., Salas, M., and Beyer, C. (1969) Effect of estrogen on the responsivity of hypothalamic and mesencephalic neurons in the female cat. *Brain Res., 15:* 439–446.

Altman, J., and Bayer, S. A. (1978a) Development of the diencephalon in the rat. I. Autoradiographic study of the time of origin and settling patterns of neurons of the hypothalamus. *J. Comp. Neurol., 182:* 945–972.

Altman, J., and Bayer, S. A. (1978b) Development of the diencephalon in the rat. II. Correlation of the embryonic development of the hypothalamus with the time of origin of its neurons. *J. Comp. Neurol., 182:* 973–994.

Altman, J., and Bayer, S. A. (1978c) Development of the diencephalon in the rat. III. Ontogeny of the specialized ventricular linings of the hypothalamic third ventricle. *J. Comp. Neurol., 182:* 995–1016.

Amoss, M., Blackwell, R., and Guillemin, R. (1972) Stimulation of ovulation in the rabbit triggered by synthetic LRF. *J. Clin. Endocrinol. Metab., 34:* 434–436.

Amoss, M., Burgus, R., Blackwell, R., Vale, W., Fellows, R., and Guillemin, R. (1971) Purification, amino acid composition and n-terminus of the hypothalamic luteinizing hormone releasing factor (LRF) of ovine origin. *Biochem. Biophys. Res. Commun., 44:* 205–210.

Anderson, F. D., and Berry, C. M. (1959) Degeneration studies of long ascending fiber systems in the cat brain stem. *J. Comp. Neurol., 111:* 195–229.

Anderson, J. N., Peck, E. J., Jr., and Clark, J. H. (1975) Estrogen-induced uterine responses and growth: relationship to receptor estrogen binding by uterine nuclei. *Endocrinology, 96:* 160–167.

Antonetty, C. M., and Webster, K. E. (1975) The organization of the spinotectal projection. An experimental study in the rat. *J. Comp. Neurol., 163:* 449–466.

Applebaum, A. E., Beall, J. E., Foreman, R. D., and Willis, W. D. (1975) Organization and receptive fields of primate spinothalamic tract neurons. *J. Neurophysiol., 38:* 572–586.

Arai, Y., and Gorski, R. A. (1968) Effect of anti-estrogen on steroid induced sexual receptivity in ovariectomized rats. *Physiol. Behav., 3:* 351–353.

Araki, S., Ferin, M., Zimmerman, E. A., and Vande Wiele, R. L. (1975) Ovarian modulation of immunoreactive gonadotropins-releasing hormone (Gn-RH) in the rat brain: evidence for a differential effect on the anterior and midhypothalamus. *Endocrinology, 96:* 644–650.

Arimura, A., Matsuo, H., Baba, Y., Debeljuk, L., Sandow, J., and Schally, A. V. (1972) Stimulation of release of LH by synthetic LH-RH *in vivo:* I. A comparative study of natural and synthetic hormones. *Endocrinology, 90:* 163–168.

Arnold, A., Nottebohm, F., and Pfaff, D. W. (1976) Hormone-concentrating cells in vocal control and other areas of the brain of the zebra finch (*Poephila guttata*). *J. Comp. Neurol., 165:* 487–512.

Averill, R. L. W., and Purves, H. D. (1963) Differential effects of permanent hypothalamic lesions on reproduction and lactation in rats. *J. Endocrinol., 26:* 463–477.

Bagshaw, R. J., Iizuka, M., and Peterson, L. H. (1971) Effect of interaction of the hypothalamus and the carotid sinus mechanoreceptor system on renal hemodynamics in the anesthetized dog. *Circ. Res., 29:* 569–585.

Ball, J. (1934) Sex behavior of the rat after removal of the uterus and vagina. *J. Comp. Psychol., 18:* 419–422.

Bard, P. (1939) Central nervous mechanisms for emotional behavior patterns in animals. *Res. Publ. Assoc. Res. Nerv. Ment. Dis., 19:* 190–218.

Barfield, R. J. (1976) Activation of estrous behavior by intracerebral implants of estradiol benzoate (EB) in ovariectomized rats. *Fed. Proc., 35:* 429.

Barfield, R. J., and Chen, J. J. (1977) Activation of estrous behavior in ovariectomized rats by intracerebral implants of estradiol benzoate. *Endocrinology, 101:* 1716–1725.

Barfield, R. J., Ronay, G., and Pfaff, D. W. (1978) Autoradiographic localization of androgen-concentrating cells in the brain of the male domestic fowl. *Neuroendocrinology, 26:* 297–311.

Barraclough, C. A., and Gorski, R. A. (1961) Evidence that the hypothalamus is responsible for androgen-induced sterility in the female rat. *Endocrinology, 68:* 68–76.

Basbaum, A. I., Clanton, C. H., and Fields, H. L. (1976) Ascending projections of nucleus gigantocellularis and nucleus raphe magnus in the cat. An autoradiographic study. *Anat. Rec., 184:* 354.

Bateson, G. (1979) *Mind and Nature: A Necessary Unity.* New York: Dutton.

Bayliss, W. M. (1920) *Principles of General Physiology,* third edition. London: Putnam.

Beach, F. A. (1942) Importance of progesterone to induction of sexual receptivity in spayed female rats. *Proc. Soc. Exp. Biol. Med., 51:* 369–371.

Beach, F. A. (1944) Effects of injury to the cerebral cortex upon sexually receptive behavior in the female rat. *Psychosom. Med., 6:* 40–55.

Beach, F. A. (1948) *Hormones and Behavior.* New York: Hoeber.

Beach, F. A., and Orndorff, R. K. (1974) Variation in the responsiveness of female rats to ovarian hormones as a function of preceding hormonal depri-vation. *Horm. Behav., 5:* 202–205.

Bermant, G., and Westbrook, W. (1966) Peripheral factors in the regulation of sexual contact by female rats. *J. Comp. Physiol. Psychol., 61:* 244–250.

Blandau, R. J., Boling, J. L., and Young, W. C. (1941) The length of heat in the albino rat as determined by the copulatory response. *Anat. Rec., 79:* 453–463.

Brawer, J. R., and Sonnenschein, C. (1975) Cytopathological effects of estradiol on the arcuate nucleus of the female rat. A possible mechanism for pituitary tumorigenesis. *Am. J. Anat., 144:* 57–88.

Brickman, A. L., Calaresu, F. R., and Mogenson, G. J. (1979) Bradycardia during stimulation of the septum and somatic afferents in the rabbit. *Am. J. Physiol., 236:* R225–R230.

Brink, E., Modianos, D., and Pfaff, D. W. (1979) Ablations of epaxial deep back muscles. Effects on lordosis behavior in the female rat. *Brain Behav. Evol., 17:* 67–88.

Brink, E., and Pfaff, D. W. (1979a) Vertebral muscles of the back and tail in the rat. *Brain Behav. Evol., 17:* 1–47.

Brink, E., and Pfaff, D. W. (1979b) Supraspinal and segmental influence on medial and lateral longissimus nerve activity in rats. *Soc. Neurosci. Abstr., 5:* 364 (Abstract 1214).

Brink, E., and Pfaff, D. W. (1980) Descending influences on lumbar epaxial motoneurons in the rat. To be submitted for publication.

Brink, E .E., Morrell, J. I., and Pfaff, D. W. (1979) Localization of lumbar epaxial motoneurons in the rat. *Brain Res., 170:* 23–41.

Brodal, A. (1969) *Neurological Anatomy.* New York: Oxford University Press.

Brodal, A., Pompeiano, O., and Walberg, F. (1962) *The Vestibular Nuclei and Their Connections, Anatomy and Functional Correlations.* Springfield, Ill.: Thomas.

Brookhart, J. M., Dey, F. L., and Ranson, S. W. (1940) Failure of ovarian hormones to cause mating reactions in spayed guinea pigs with hypothalamic lesions. *Proc. Soc. Exp. Biol. Med., 44:* 61–64.

Brookhart, J. M., Dey, F. L., and Ranson, S. W. (1941) The abolition of mating behavior by hypothalamic lesions in guinea pigs. *Endocrinology, 28:* 561–565.

Brown, L. T. (1974) Rubrospinal projections in the rat. *J. Comp. Neurol., 154:* 169–188.

Bueno, J., and Pfaff, D. W. (1976) Single unit recording in hypothalamus and preoptic area of estrogen-treated and untreated ovariectomized female rats. *Brain Res., 101:* 67–78.

Buller, R. E., and O'Malley, B. W. (1976) The biology and mechanism of steroid hormone interactions with the eukaryotic nucleus. *Biochem. Pharmacol., 25:* 1–12.

Burgess, P. R., and Perl, G. R. (1973) Cutaneous mechanoreceptors and noci-ceptors. In A. Iggo (Ed.), *Somatosensory System, Handbook of Sensory Physiology, Vol. II.* New York: Springer-Verlag, pp. 29–78.

Burgess, P. R., Petit, D., and Warren, R. M. (1968) Receptor types in cat hairy skin supplied by myelinated fibers. *J. Neurophysiol., 31:* 833–848.

Burgus, R., Butcher, M., Amoss, M., Ling, N., Monahan, M., Rivier, J., Fellows, R., Blackwell, R., Vale, W., and Guillemin, R. (1972) Primary structure of the ovine hypothalamic luteinizing hormone-releasing factor (LRF). *Proc. Natl. Acad. Sci. U.S.A., 69:* 278–282.

Burgus, R., Butcher, M., Ling, N., Monahan, M., Rivier, J., Fellows, R.,

Amoss, M., Blackwell, R., Vale, W., and Guillemin, R. (1971) Structure moléculaire du facteur hypothalamique (LRF) d'origine ovine contrôlant la sécrétion de l'hormone gonadotrope hypophysaire de lutéinisation (LH). *C.R. Acad. Sci. (Paris) [D], 273:* 1611–1613.

Caggiula, A. R. (1970) Analysis of the copulation-reward properties of posterior hypothalamic stimulation in male rats. *J. Comp. Physiol. Psychol., 70:* 399–412.

Caggiula, A. R., Antelman, S. M., and Zigmond, M. J. (1973) Disruption of copulation in male rats after hypothalamic lesions: a behavioral, anatomical and neurochemical analysis. *Brain Res., 59:* 273–287.

Caggiula, A. R., Gay, V. L., Antelman, S. M., and Leggens, J. (1975) Disruption of copulation in male rats after hypothalamic lesions: a neuroendocrine analysis. *Neuroendocrinology, 17:* 193–202.

Caggiula, A. R., and Hoebel, B. G. (1966) "Copulation-reward site" in the posterior hypothalamus. *Science, 153:* 1284–1285.

Calaresu, F. R. (1974) Central pathways of integration of cardiovascular responses. XXVI International Congress of Physiological Sciences, New Delhi, p. 21.

Capony, E., and Rochefort, H. (1975) In vivo effect of anti-estrogens on the localisation and replenishment of estrogen receptor. *Mol. Cell. Endocrinol., 3:* 233–251.

Carrer, H., Asch, G., and Aron, C. (1973) New facts concerning the role played by the ventromedial nucleus in the control of estrous cycle duration and sexual receptivity in the rat. *Neuroendocrinology, 13:* 129–138.

Carrer, H. F. (1978) Mesencephalic participation in the control of sexual behavior in the female rat. *J. Comp. Physiol. Psychol., 92:* 877–887.

Chambers, W. F., and Howe, G. (1968) A study of estrogen-sensitive hypothalamic centers using a technique for rapid application and removal of estradiol. *Proc. Soc. Exp. Biol. Med., 128:* 292–294.

Chan, S. H. H., and Barnes, C. D. (1972) A presynaptic mechanism evoked from brain stem reticular formation in the lumbar cord and its temporal significance. *Brain Res., 45:* 101–114.

Chazal, G., Faudon, M., Gogan, E., and Rotsztejn, W. (1975) Effects of two estradiol antagonists upon the estradiol uptake in the rat brain and peripheral tissues. *Brain Res., 89:* 245–254.

Chen, H. I., and Chai, C. Y. (1974) Pulmonary edema and hemorrhage as a consequence of systemic vasoconstriction. *Am. J. Physiol., 227:* 144–151.

Chi, C. C. (1970) An experimental silver study of the ascending projections of the central gray substance and adjacent tegmentum in the rat with observations in the cat. *J. Comp. Neurol., 139:* 259–272.

Christensen, L. W., and Gorski, R. A. (1976) Sites of neonatal gonadal steroid action in hypothalamic sexual differentiation. V International Congress of Endocrinology, Hamburg, Abstract 217, p. 88.

Ciaccio, L. A., and Lisk, R. D. (1973) Central control of estrous behavior in the female golden hamster. *Neuroendocrinology, 13:* 21–28.

Ciriello, J., Calaresu, F. R., and Mogenson, G. J. (1975) Neural pathways mediating cardiovascular responses elicited by stimulation of the septum in the rat. Society for Neuroscience, Abstract 655, p. 422.

Clark, G. (1942) Sexual behavior in rats with lesions in the anterior hypothalamus. *Am. J. Physiol., 137:* 746–749.

Clegg, M. T., Santolucito, J. A., Smith, J. D., and Ganong, W. F. (1958) The effect of hypothalamic lesions on sexual behavior and estrous cycles in the ewe. *Endocrinology, 62:* 790–797.

Clemens, J. A. Smalstig, E. B., and Sawyer, B. D. (1976) Studies on the role of the preoptic area in the control of reproductive function in the rat. *Endocrinology, 99:* 728–735.

Clemens, L. G., Wallen, K., and Gorski, R. A. (1969) Mating behavior: facilitation in the female rat after cortical application of potassium chloride. *Science, 157:* 1208–1209.

Cohen, R., and Pfaff, D. W. (1979) Ultrastructure of neurons of the ventromedial nucleus of ovariectomized and estrogen-treated female rats. *Soc. Neurosci. Abstr., 5:* 230 (Abstract 747).

Conrad, L., Leonard, C., and Pfaff, D. W. (1974) Connections of the median and dorsal raphe nuclei in the rat: an autoradiographic and degeneration study. *J. Comp. Neurol., 156:* 179–206.

Conrad, L. A., and Pfaff, D. W. (1975) Axonal projections of medial preoptic and anterior hypothalamic neurons. *Science, 190:* 1112–1114.

Conrad, L. C. A., and Pfaff, D. W. (1976a) Autoradiographic study of efferents from medial basal forebrain and hypothalamus in the rat. I. Medial preoptic area. *J. Comp. Neurol., 169:* 185–220.

Conrad, L. C. A., and Pfaff, D. W. (1976b) Autoradiographic study of efferents from medial basal forebrain and hypothalamus in the rat. II. Medial anterior hypothalamus. *J. Comp. Neurol., 169:* 221–262.

Conrad, L. C. A., and Pfaff, D. W. (1976c) Autoradiographic tracing of nucleus accumbens efferents in the rat. *Brain Res., 113:* 589–596.

Conrad, L. C. A., and Pfaff, D. W. (1977) Hypothalamic neuroanatomy: steroid hormone binding and axonal projections. In G. Bourne (Ed.), *International Review of Cytology*. New York: Academic Press.

Cook, W. A., Jr., Cangiano, A., and Pompeiano, O. (1969a) Dorsal root potentials in the lumbar cord evoked from the vestibular system. *Arch. Ital. Biol., 107:* 275–295.

Cook, W. A., Jr., Cangiano, A., and Pompeiano, O. (1969b) Vestibular control of transmission in primary afferents to the lumbar spinal cord. *Arch. Ital. Biol., 107:* 296–320.

Cowan, W. M., Gottelieb, D. I., Hendrickson, A. E., Price, J. L., and Woolsey, T. A. (1972) The autoradiographic demonstration of axonal connections in the central nervous system. *Brain Res., 37:* 21–51.

Creed, R. S., Denny-Brown, D., Eccles, J. C., Liddell, E. G. T., and Sherrington, C. S. (1932) *Reflex Activity of the Spinal Cord*. Oxford: Clarendon Press.

Crews, D., and Silver, R. (1980) In R. Goy and D. W. Pfaff (Eds.), *Neurobiology of Reproduction*. New York: Plenum.

Cross, B. A., and Dyer, R. G. (1971) Cyclic changes in neurons of the anterior hypothalamus during the rat estrous cycle and the effect of anesthesia. In C. H. Sawyer and R. A. Gorski (Eds.), *Steroid Hormones and Brain Function, UCLA Forum in Medical Sciences, No. 15*. Los Angeles: University of California Press, pp. 95–102.

Cross, B. A., and Dyer, R. G. (1972) Ovarian modulation of unit activity in the anterior hypothalamus of the cyclic rat. *J. Physiol. (Lond.), 222:* 25P.

Davidson, J. M. (1966) Activation of the male rat's sexual behavior by intracerebral implantation of androgen. *Endocrinology, 79:* 783–794.

Davidson, J. M., Rodgers, C. H., Smith, E. R., and Bloch, G. J. (1968) Stimulation of female sex behavior in adrenalectomized rats with estrogen alone. *Endocrinology, 82:* 193–195.

Davis, P., Krieger, M., and Pfaff, D. (1980) Manuscript in preparation.

Davis, P. G., McEwen, B., and Pfaff, D. W. (1979) Localized behavioral effects of tritiated estradiol implants in the ventromedial hypothalamus of female rats. *Endocrinology, 104:* 898–903.

Davis, R. E., Morrell, J. I., and Pfaff, D. W. (1977) Autoradiographic localization of sex steroid-concentrating cells in the brain of the teleost *Macropodus opercularis* (Osteichthyes: Belontiidae). *Gen. Comp. Endocrinol., 33:* 496–505.

Dempsey, E. W., and Rioch, D. McK. (1939) The localization in the brain stem of the oestrous responses of the female guinea pig. *J. Neurophysiol., 2:* 9–18.

Dertouzos, M. L. (1965) *Threshold Logic: A Synthesis Approach.* Research Monograph No. 32. Cambridge, Mass.: M.I.T. Press.

Dey, F. L. (1941) Changes in ovaries and uteri in guinea pigs with hypothalamic lesions. *Am. J. Anat., 69:* 61–87.

Dey, F. L., Fisher, C., Berry, C. M., and Ranson, S. W. (1940) Disturbances in reproductive functions caused by hypothalamic lesions in female guinea pigs. *Am. J. Physiol., 129:* 39–46.

Dey, F. L., Leininger, C. R., and Ranson, S. W. (1942) The effect of hypophysial lesions on mating behavior in female guinea pigs. *Endocrinology, 30:* 323–326.

Diakow, C., Pfaff, D. W., and Komisaruk, B. (1973) Sensory and hormonal interactions in eliciting lordosis. *Fed. Proc., 32:* 241 (Abstr.).

Dilly, P. N., Wall, P. D., and Webster, K. E. (1968) Cells of origin of the spinothalamic tract in the cat and rat. *Exp. Neurol., 21:* 550–562.

Djojosugito, A. M., Folkow, B., Kylstra, P. H., Lisander, B., and Tuttle, R. S. (1970) Differentiated interactions between the hypothalamic defence reaction and baroreceptor reflexes. I. Effects on heart rate and regional flow resistance. *Acta Physiol. Scand., 78:* 376–385.

Domanski, E., Przekop, F., and Skubiszewski, B. (1972) The role of the anterior regions of the medial basal hypothalamus in the control of ovulation and sexual behavior in sheep. *Acta Neurobiol. Exp., 32:* 753–762.

Dörner, G., Döcke, F., and Gotz, F. (1975) Male-like sexual behaviour of female rats with unilateral lesions in the hypothalamic ventromedial nuclear region. *Endokrinologie, 65:* 133–137.

Dörner, G., Döcke, F., and Hinz, G. (1969) Homo- and hypersexuality in rats with hypothalamic lesions. *Neuroendocrinology, 4:* 20–24.

Dörner, G., Döcke, F., and Moustafa, S. (1968) Differential localization of a male and a female hypothalamic mating centre. *J. Reprod. Fertil., 17:* 583–586.

Dyer, R. G. (1973) An electrophysiological dissection of the hypothalamic regions which regulate the pre-ovulatory secretion of luteinizing hormone in the rat. *J. Physiol. (Lond.), 234:* 421–442.

Dyer, R. G., and Burnet, F. (1976) Effects of ferrous ions on preoptic area neurones and luteinizing hormone secretion in the rat. *J. Endocrinol., 69:* 247–254.

Dyer, R. G., Pritchett, C. J., and Cross, B. A. (1972) Unit activity in the diencephalon of female rats during the oestrous cycle. *J. Endocrinol., 53:* 151–160.

Ebbesson, S. O. E. (1967) Ascending axon degeneration following hemisection of the spinal cord in the tegu lizard (*Tupinambis nigropunctatus*). *Brain Res., 5:* 178–206.

Ebbesson, S. O. E. (1969) Brain stem afferents from the spinal cord in a sample of reptilian and amphibian species. *Ann. N. Y. Acad. Sci., 167:* 80–101.

Eccles, J. C., Nicoll, R. A., Rantucci, T., Taborikova, H., and Willey, T. J. (1976) Topographic studies on medial reticular nucleus. *J. Neurophysiol., 39:* 109–118.

Eccles, J. C., Nicoll, R. A., Schwarz, D. W. F., Taborikova, H., and Willey, T. J. (1975) Reticulospinal neurons with and without monosynaptic inputs from cerebellar nuclei. *J. Neurophysiol., 38:* 513–530.

Eccles, J. C., Nicoll, R. A., Taborikova, H., and Willey, T. J. (1975) Medial reticular neurons projecting rostrally. *J. Neurophysiol., 38:* 531–538.

Eccles, R. M., and Lundberg, A. (1959) Supraspinal control in motoneurones mediating spinal reflexes. *J. Physiol., 147:* 565–584.

Edwards, D. A., and Mathews, D. (1977) The ventromedial nucleus of the hypothalamus and the hormonal arousal of sexual behaviors in the female rat. *Physiol. Behav., in press.*

Edwards, D. A., and Warner, P. (1972) Olfactory bulb removal facilitates the hormonal induction of sexual receptivity in the female rat. *Horm. Behav., 3:* 321–332.

Edwards, S. B. (1975) Autoradiographic studies of the projections of the midbrain reticular formation: descending projections of nucleus cuneiformis. *J. Comp. Neurol., 161:* 341–358.

Edwards, S. B., and de Olmos, J. S. (1976) Autoradiographic studies of the projections of the midbrain reticular formation: ascending projections of nucleus cuneiformis. *J. Comp. Neurol., 165:* 417–432.

Egger, M. D., and Wall, P. D. (1971) The plantar cushion reflex circuit: An oligosynaptic cutaneous reflex. *J. Physiol. (Lond.), 216:* 483–501.

Eibergen, R. D., and Caggiula, A. R. (1973) Ventral midbrain involvement in copulatory behavior of the male rat. *Physiol. Behav., 10:* 435–442.

Eisenfeld, A. J., and Axelrod, J. (1965) Selectivity of estrogen distribution in tissues. *J. Pharmacol. Exp. Ther., 150:* 469–475.

Eisenfeld, A. J., and Axelrod, J. (1966) Effect of steroid hormones, ovariectomy, estrogen pretreatment, sex and immaturity on the distribution of ^{3}H-estradiol. *Endocrinology, 79:* 38–42.

Engberg, I. (1964) Reflexes to foot muscles in the cat. *Acta Physiol. Scand., 52 (Suppl. 235):* 1–64.

Everett, J. W. (1969) Neuroendocrine aspects of mammalian reproduction. *Ann. Rev. Physiol., 31:* 383–416.

Ewald, J. R. (1892) *Physiologische Untersuchungen über das Endorgan des N. Oktavus.* Bergmann: Wiesbaden. Cited in Meyer, D. L., and Bullock, T. H. (1977) The hypothesis of sense-organ-dependent tonus mechanisms: History of a concept. In B. Wenzel and P. Ziegler (Eds.), *Tonic Functions of Sensory Systems. Ann. N. Y. Acad. Sci., 290:* 3–17.

Fearing, F. (1930) *Reflex Action.* Baltimore: Williams & Wilkins.

Feder, H. H. (1980) Chapter in R. Goy and D. W. Pfaff (Eds.), *Neurobiology of Reproduction.* New York: Plenum, in press.

Feder, H. H., Brown-Grant, K., and Corker, C. S. (1971) Pre-ovulatory progesterone, the adrenal cortex and the 'critical period' for luteinizing hormone release in rats. *J. Endocrinol., 50:* 29–39.

Floody, O., and Pfaff, D. W. (1974) Steroid hormones and aggressive behavior:

approaches to the study of hormone-sensitive brain mechanisms for behavior. *Res. Publ. Assoc. Res. Nerv. Ment. Dis. 52:* 149–185.

Floody, O. R., and Pfaff, D. W. (1977a) Communication among hamsters by high-frequency acoustic signals. I. Physical characteristics of hamster calls. *J. Comp. Physiol. Psychol., 91:* 794–806.

Floody, O. R., and Pfaff, D. W. (1977b) Communication among hamsters by high-frequency acoustic signals. III. Responses evoked by natural and synthetic ultrasounds. *J. Comp. Physiol. Psychol., 91:* 820–829.

Floody, O. R., Pfaff, D. W., and Lewis, C. D. (1977) Communication among hamsters by high-frequency acoustic signals: II. Determinants of calling by females and males. *J. Comp. Physiol. Psychol., 91:* 807–819.

Foreman, R. D., Hancock, M. B., and Willis, W. D. (1975) Convergence of visceral and cutaneous input onto spinothalamic tract neurons in the thoracic spinal cord of the rhesus monkey. *Society for Neuroscience,* Abstract 233, p. 148.

Fox, J. E. (1970) Reticulospinal neurones in the rat. *Brain Res., 23:* 35–40.

Gerall, A. A., and Dunlap, J. L. (1973) The effect of experience and hormones on the initial receptivity in female and male rats. *Physiol. Behav., 10:* 851–854.

Gerlach, J., McEwen, B., Pfaff, D., Moskovitz, S., Ferin, M., Carmel, P., and Zimmerman, E. (1976) Cells in regions of rhesus monkey brain and pituitary retain radioactive estradiol, corticosterone and cortisol differentially. *Brain Res., 103:* 603–612.

Goldberg, J. M., and Moore, R. Y. (1967) Ascending projections of the lateral lemniscus in the cat and monkey. *J. Comp. Neurol., 129:* 143–156.

Goy, R. W., and Phoenix, C. H. (1963) Hypothalamic regulation of female sexual behaviour; establishment of behavioural oestrus in spayed guinea-pigs following hypothalamic lesions. *J. Reprod. Fertil., 5:* 23–40.

Graybiel, A. M. (1973) The thalamo-cortical projection of the so-called posterior nuclear group: a study with anterograde degeneration methods in the cat. *Brain Res., 49:* 229–244.

Green, R., Luttge, W. G., and Whalen, R. E. (1970) Induction of receptivity in ovariectomized female rats by a single intravenous injection of estradiol-17β. *Physiol. Behav., 5:* 137–141.

Greer, M. A. (1953) The effect of progesterone on persistent vaginal estrus produced by hypothalamic lesions in the rat. *Endocrinology, 53:* 380–390.

Grillner, S., Hongo, T., and Lund, S. (1968) The origin of descending fibres monosynaptically activating spinoreticular neurones. *Brain Res., 10:* 259–262.

Grillner, S., Hongo, T., and Lund, S. (1970) The vestibulospinal tract. Effects on alpha-motoneurones in the lumbosacral spinal cord in the cat. *Exp. Brain Res., 10:* 94–120.

Grillner, S., Hongo, T., and Lund, S. (1971) Convergent effects on alpha motoneurones from the vestibulospinal tract and a pathway descending in the medial longitudinal fasciculus. *Exp. Brain Res., 12:* 457–479.

Hagamen, W. D., and Brooks, D. C. (1958) Sexual behavior of female cats following lesions of the ventromedial nucleus of the hypothalamus. *Anat. Rec., 130:* 414 (Abstr. 348).

Halasz, B. (1969) The endocrine effects of isolation of the hypothalamus from the rest of the brain. In W. F. Ganong and L. Martini (Eds.), *Frontiers in Neuroendocrinology, 1969.* New York: Oxford University Press, pp. 307–342.

Halasz, B., and Gorski, R. A. (1967) Gonadotrophic hormone secretion in female rats after partial or total interruption of neural afferents to the medial basal hypothalamus. *Endocrinology, 80:* 608–622.

Halpern, M. H., Morrell, J., and Pfaff, D. W. (1980) Autoradiography of sex hormone concentrating cells in the brain of the garter snake. *Endocrine Soc. Abstr.,* in press.

Hamilton, B. L. (1972) Projections of the subnuclear areas of the periaqueductal gray matter in the cat. *Society for Neuroscience* Abstract 112, p. 148.

Hamilton, B. L., and Skultety, F. M. (1970) Efferent connections of the periaqueductal gray matter in the cat. *J. Comp. Neurol., 139:* 105–114.

Hard, E., and Larsson, K. (1968) Effects of mounts without intromission upon sexual behavior in male rats. *Anim. Behav., 16:* 538–540.

Hardy, D. F., and DeBold, J. F. (1971) Effects of mounts without intromission upon the behavior of female rats during the onset of estrogen-induced heat. *Physiol. Behav. 7:* 643–645.

Hart, B. L. (1969) Gonadal hormones and sexual reflexes in the female rat. *Horm. Behav., 1:* 65–71.

Hassen, A. H., and Barnes, C. D. (1975) Bilateral effects of vestibular nerve stimulation on activity in the lumbar spinal cord. *Brain Res., 90:* 221–233.

Hayle, T. H. (1973) A comparative study of spinal projections to the brain (except cerebellum) in three classes of poikilothermic vertebrates. *J. Comp. Neurol., 149:* 463–476.

Heath, C. J., and Jones, E. G. (1971) An experimental study of ascending connections from the posterior group of thalamic nuclei in the cat. *J. Comp. Neurol., 141:* 397–426.

Hendrickson, A. (1975) Tracing neuronal connections with radioisotopes applied extracellularly. *Fed. Proc., 34:* 1612–1615.

Herndon, J. G., and Neill, D. B. (1973) Amphetamine reversal of sexual impairment following anterior hypothalamic lesions in female rats. *Pharmacol. Biochem. Behav., 1:* 285–288.

Herrick, C. J., and Bishop, G. H. (1958) A comparative survey of the spinal lemniscus systems. In H. H. Jasper, L. D. Proctor, R. S. Knighton, W. C. Noshay, and R. T. Costello (Eds.), *Reticular Formation of the Brain.* Boston: Little, Brown, pp. 353–360.

Hess, W. R. (1954) *Diencephalon. Autonomic and Extrapyramidal Functions.* New York: Grune & Stratton.

Hess, W. R. (1957) *The Functional Organization of the Diencephalon.* New York: Grune & Stratton.

Hill, F. J., and Peterson, G. R. (1974) *Introduction to Switching Theory and Logical Design,* second edition. New York: Wiley.

Hilton, S. M., and Spyer, K. M. (1971) Participation of the anterior hypothalamus in the baroreceptor reflex. *J. Physiol., 218:* 271–293.

Hitt, J. C., Bryon, D. M., and Modianos, D. T. (1973) Effects of rostral medial forebrain bundle and olfactory tubercle lesions upon sexual behavior of male rats. *J. Comp. Physiol. Psychol., 82:* 30–36.

Hitt, J. C., Hendricks, S. E., Ginsberg, S. I., and Lewis, J. H. (1970) Disruption of male, but not female, sexual behavior in rats by medial forebrain bundle lesions. *J. Comp. Physiol. Psychol., 73:* 377–384.

Holmqvist, B., Lundberg, A., and Oscarsson, O. (1960a) A supraspinal control system monosynaptically connected with an ascending spinal pathway. *Arch. Ital. Biol., 98:* 402–422

Holmqvist, B., Lundberg, A., and Oscarsson, O. (1960b) Supraspinal inhibitory control of transmission to three ascending spinal pathways influenced by the flexion reflex afferents. *Arch. Ital. Biol., 98:* 60–80.

Hongo, T., Kudo, N., and Tanaka, R. (1975) The vestibulospinal tract: crossed and uncrossed effects on hindlimb motoneurones in the cat. *Exp. Brain Res., 24:* 37–55.

Horn, G., and Hill, R. M. (1966) Responsiveness to sensory stimulation of units in the superior colliculus and subjacent tecto-tegmental regions of the rabbit. *Exp. Neurol., 14:* 199–223.

Hornby, J. B., and Rose, J. D. (1976) Responses of caudal brain stem neurons to vaginal and somatosensory stimulation in the rat and evidence of genital–nociceptive interactions. *Exp. Neurol., 51:* 363–376.

Hough, J. C., Jr., Ho, G. K-W, Cooke, P. H., and Quadagno, D. M. (1974) Actinomycin D: reversible inhibition of lordosis behavior and correlated changes in nucleolar morphology. *Horm. Behav., 5:* 367–375.

Houk, J. C. (1979) Regulation of stiffness by skeletomotor reflexes. *Ann. Rev. Physiol., 41:* 99–114.

Huber, F. (1978) The insect nervous system and insect behaviour. *Anim. Behav., 26:* 969–981.

Iggo, A. (1966) Cutaneous receptors with a high sensitivity to mechanical displacement. In A. V. S. de Reuck and J. Knight (Eds.), *Touch, Heat and Pain.* Boston: Little, Brown, pp. 237–256.

James, W. (1890) *The Principles of Psychology,* Vol. 1. New York: Holt. (Dover edition, 1950, p. 23).

Job, C. (1953) Ueber autogene Inhition und Reflexumkehr bei spinalisierten und decerebrierten Katzen. *Pfluegers Arch., 256:* 406–418.

Johnston, P., and Davidson, J. M. (1972) Intracerebral androgens and sexual behavior in the male rat. *Horm. Behav., 3:* 345–357.

Kalra, S. P., and Sawyer, C. H. (1970) Blockade of copulation-induced ovulation in the rat by anterior hypothalamic deafferentation. *Endocrinology, 87:* 1124–1128.

Kato, J., and Villee, C. A. (1967a) Factors affecting uptake of estradiol-6,7-^{3}H by the hypophysis and hypothalamus. *Endocrinology, 80:* 1113–1138.

Kato, J., and Villee, C. A. (1967b) Preferential uptake of estradiol by the anterior hypothalamus of the rat. *Endocrinology, 80:* 567–575.

Katzenellenbogen, B. S., and Ferguson, E. R. (1975) Antiestrogen action in the uterus: biological ineffectiveness of nuclear bound estradiol after antiestrogen. *Endocrinology, 97:* 1–12.

Kaufman, R. S. (1953) Effects of preventing intromission upon sexual behavior of rats. *J. Comp. Physiol. Psychol., 46:* 209–211.

Kawakami, M., and Sawyer, C. H. (1959a) Induction of behavioral and electroencephalographic changes in the rabbit by hormone administration and brain stimulation. *Endocrinology, 65:* 631–643.

Kawakami, M., and Sawyer, C. H. (1959b) Neuroendocrine correlates of changes in brain activity thresholds by sex steroids and pituitary hormones. *Endocrinology, 65:* 652–668.

Kawakami, M., Terasawa, E., and Ibuki, T. (1970) Changes in multiple unit activity of the brain during the estrous cycle. *Neuroendocrinology, 6:* 30–48.

Kawakami, M., Terasawa, E., Ibuki, T., and Manaka, M. (1971) Effects of sex hormones and ovulation-blocking steroids and drugs on electrical activity of the rat brain. In C. H. Sawyer and R. A. Gorski (Eds.), *Steroid Hormones and Brain Function, UCLA Forum in Medical Sciences, No. 15*. Los Angeles: University of California Press, pp. 79–93.

Kelley, D. B., Lieberburg, I., McEwen, B. S., and Pfaff, D. W. (1978) Autoradiographic and biochemical studies of steroid hormone-concentrating cells in the brain of *Rana pipiens*. *Brain Res., 140:* 287–305.

Kelley, D. B., Morrell, J. I., and Pfaff, D. W. (1975) Autoradiographic localization of hormone-concentrating cells in the brain of an amphibian, *Xenopus laevis*. I. Testosterone. *J. Comp. Neurol., 164:* 47–62.

Kelley, D. B., and Pfaff, D. W. (1975) Locations of steroid hormone-concentrating cells in the central nervous system of *Rana pipiens*. *Society for Neuroscience,* Abstract 681, p. 438.

Kelley, D. B., and Pfaff, D. W. (1976) Hormone effects on male sex behavior in adult South African clawed frogs, *Xenopus laevis*. *Horm. Behav., 7:* 159–182.

Kelley, D. B., and Pfaff, D. W. (1978) Generalizations from comparative studies on neuroanatomical and endocrine mechanisms of sexual behaviour. In J. Hutchison (Ed.), *Biological Determinants of Sexual Behavior*. Chicester, England: Wiley, pp. 225–254.

Kelly, M. J., Moss, R. L., and Dudley, C. A. (1976) Differential sensitivity of preoptic–septal neurons to microelectrophoresed estrogen during the estrous cycle. *Brain Res., 114:* 152–157.

Kennedy, G. C. (1964) Hypothalamic control of the endocrine and behavioural changes associated with oestrus in the rat. *J. Physiol., 172:* 383–392.

Kennedy, G. C., and Mitra, J. (1963) Hypothalamic control of energy balance and the reproductive cycle in the rat. *J. Physiol., 166:* 395–407.

Kimble, D. D., Rogers, L., and Hendrickson, C. W. (1967) Hippocampal lesions disrupt maternal, not sexual, behavior in the albino rat. *J. Comp. Physiol. Psychol., 63:* 401–407.

King, J. C., Williams, T. H., and Gerall, A. A. (1974) Transformations of hypothalamic arcuate neurons. I. Changes associated with stages of the estrous cycle. *Cell Tissue Res., 153:* 497–515.

Kohavi, Z. (1978) *Switching and Finite Automata Theory,* second edition. New York: McGraw-Hill.

Koizumi, K., Nishino, H., and Colman, D. (1975) The suprachiasmatic nuclei and circadian rhythms. *Society for Neuroscience,* Abstract 692, p. 446.

Komisaruk, B. R., Adler, N. T., and Hutchison, J. (1972) Genital sensory field: enlargement by estrogen treatment in female rats. *Science, 178:* 1295–1298.

Komisaruk, B. R., and Diakow, C. (1973) Lordosis reflex intensity in rats in relation to the estrous cycle, ovariectomy, estrogen administration and mating behavior. *Endocrinology, 93:* 548–557.

Kow, L.-M., Grill, H., and Pfaff, D. W. (1978) Elimination of lordosis in decerebrate female rats: observations from acute and chronic prepartions. *Physiol. Behav., 20:* 171–174.

Kow, L.-M., Malsbury, C. W., and Pfaff, D. W. (1974a) Effects of medial hypothalamic lesions on the lordosis response in female hamsters. *Proc. Soc. Neurosci.,* Abstract 365, p. 291.

Kow, L.-M., Malsbury, C., and Pfaff, D. W. (1974b) Effects of progesterone on female reproductive behavior in rats: possible modes of action and role in behavioral sex differences. In W. Montagna and W. Sadler (Eds.), *Reproductive Behavior*. New York: Plenum, pp. 179–210.

Kow, L.-M., Malsbury, C., and Pfaff, D. W. (1976) Lordosis in the male golden hamster elicited by manual stimulation: characteristics and hormonal sensitivity. *J. Comp. Physiol. Psychol., 90:* 26–40.

Kow, L.-M., Montgomery, M., and Pfaff, D. W. (1973) Spinal tract transections and the lordosis reflex in female rats. *Physiologist, 16:* 367 (Abstr.).

Kow, L.-M., Montgomery, M., and Pfaff, D. W. (1977) Effect of spinal cord transections on lordosis reflex in female rats. *Brain Res., 123:* 75–88.

Kow, L.-M., Montgomery, M. O., and Pfaff, D. W. (1979) Triggering of lordosis reflex in female rats with somatosensory stimulation: quantitative determination of stimulus parameters. *J. Neurophysiol., 42:* 195–202.

Kow, L.-M., and Pfaff, D. W. (1973) Effects of estrogen treatment on the size of receptive field and response threshold of pudendal nerve in the female rat. *Neuroendocrinology, 13:* 299–313.

Kow, L.-M., and Pfaff, D. W. (1975a) Induction of lordosis in female rats: two modes of estrogen action and the effect of adrenalectomy. *Horm. Behav., 6:* 259–276.

Kow, L.-M., and Pfaff, D. W. (1975b) Dorsal root recording relevant for mating reflexes in female rats: identification of receptive fields and effects of peripheral denervation. *J. Neurobiol., 6:* 23–37.

Kow, L.-M., and Pfaff, D. W. (1976) Sensory requirements for the lordosis reflex in female rats. *Brain Res., 101:* 47–66.

Kow, L.-M., and Pfaff, D. W. (1977) Sensory control of reproductive behavior in female rodents. In B. Wenzel and H. P. Zeigler (Eds.), *Tonic Functions of Sensory Systems. Ann. N. Y. Acad. Sci., 290:* 72–97.

Kow, L.-M., and Pfaff, D. W. (1979) Responses of single units in sixth lumbar dorsal root ganglion of female rats to mechanostimulation relevant for lordosis reflex. *J. Neurophysiol., 42:* 203–213.

Kow, L.-M., and Pfaff, D. W. (1980) Chronic recording from NGC neurons. *Experimental Brain Research,* in press.

Kow, L.-M., Zemlan, F., and Pfaff, D. W. (1980b) Pharmacologic investigations of possible lordosis components in spinal female rats. *Horm. Behav.,* in press.

Kow, L.-M., Zemlan, F., and Pfaff, D. W. (1980a) Responses of lumbosacral spinal units to mechanical stimuli related to analysis of the lordosis reflex in female rats. *J. Neurophysiol., 43:* 27–45.

Krieger, M., Conrad, L. C. A., and Pfaff, D. W. (1977) Axonal projections of neurons of ventromedial nucleus of the hypothalamus. *Anat. Rec., 187:* 770.

Krieger, M. S., Conrad, L. C. A., and Pfaff, D. W. (1979) An autoradiographic study of the efferent connections of the ventromedial nucleus of the hypothalamus. *J. Comp. Neurol., 183:* 785–816.

Krieger, M. S., Morrell, J. I., and Pfaff, D. W. (1976) Autoradiographic localization of estradiol-concentrating cells in the female hamster brain. *Neuroendocrinology, 22:* 193–205.

Krieger, M. S., and Pfaff, D. W. (1980) Projections from mesencephalic central grey in the rat. Manuscript in preparation.

Kubo, K., Mennin, S. P., and Gorski, R. A. (1975) Similarity of plasma LH release in androgenized and normal rats following electrochemical stimulation of the basal forebrain. *Endocrinology, 96:* 492–500.

Ladpli, R., and Brodal, A. (1968) Experimental studies of commissural and reticular formation projections from the vestibular nuclei in the cat. *Brain Res., 8:* 65–96.

Lan, N. C., and Katzenellenbogen, B. S. (1976) Temporal relationships between hormone receptor binding and biological response in the uterus: studies with short- and long-acting derivatives of estriol. *Endocrinology, 98:* 220–227.

Land, L. J., Reese, B. A., and Whitlock, D. G. (1975) Ascending pathways in the anterolateral funiculus of the rat spinal cord. *Society for Neuroscience,* Abstract 1058, p. 685.

La Vaque, T. J., and Rodgers, C. H. (1974) Effects of ventromedial hypothalamic lesions upon mating behavior in the female rat. *Fed. Proc., 33:* 232.

La Vaque, T. J., and Rodgers, C. H. (1975) Recovery of mating behavior in the female rat following VMH lesions. *Physiol. Behav., 14:* 59–63.

Law, T., and Meagher, W. (1958) Hypothalamic lesions and sexual behavior in the female rat. *Science, 128* 1626–1627.

Lawrence, D. G., and Kuypers, H. G. J. M. (1968a) The functional organization of the motor system in the monkey. I. The effects of bilateral pyramidal lesions. *Brain, 91:* 1–14.

Lawrence, D. G., and Kuypers, H. G. J. M. (1968a) The functional organization of the motor system of the monkey. II. The effects of lesions of the descending brain-stem pathways. *Brain, 91:* 15–36.

Liebeskind, J. C., and Mayer, D. J. (1971) Somatosensory evoked responses in the mesencephalic central gray matter of the rat. *Brain Res., 27:* 133–151.

Lincoln, D. W. (1967) Unit activity in the hypothalamus, septum and preoptic area of the rat: characteristics of spontaneous activity and the effect of oestrogen. *J. Endocrinol., 37:* 177–189.

Lincoln, D. W., and Cross, B. A. (1967) Effect of oestrogen on the responsiveness of neurones in the hypothalamus, septum and preoptic area of rats with light-induced persistent oestrus. *J. Endocrinol., 37:* 191–203.

Lindsley, D. B. (1952) Brain stem influences on spinal motor activity. *Res. Publ. Assoc. Res. Nerv. Menta. Dis., 30:* 174–195.

Lindsley, D. B., Schreiner, L. H., and Magoun, H. W. (1949) An electromyographic study of spasticity. *J. Neurophysiol., 12:* 197–205.

Lisk, R. D. (1962) Diencephalic placement of estradiol and sexual receptivity in the female rat. *Am. J. Physiol., 203:* 493–496.

Lisk, R. D. (1967) Neural localization for androgen activation of copulary behavior in the male rat. *Endocrinology, 80:* 754–761.

Lisk, R. D., and Barfield, M. A. (1975) Progesterone facilitation of sexual receptivity in rats with neural implantation of estrogen. *Neuroendocrinology, 19:* 28–35.

Lisk, R. D., Ciaccio, L. A., and Reuter, L. A. (1972) Neural centers of estrogen and progesterone action in the regulation of reproduction. In J. T. Velardo and B. A. Kasprow (Eds.), *Biology of Reproduction—Basic and Clinical Studies.* pp. 71–87.

Loeb, J. (1899) *Comparative Physiology of the Brain and Comparative Psychology.* New York: Putnam.

Loeb, J. (1912) *The Mechanistic Conception of Life.* Chicago: University of Chicago Press.

Lorenz, K. (1950) The comparative method in studying innate behaviour patterns. *Symp. Soc. Exp. Biol., 4:* 221–268.

Luine, V., and McEwen, B. S. (1980) In R. Goy and D. Pfaff (Eds.), *Neurobiology of Reproduction.* New York: Plenum.

Luine, V. N., Khylchevskaya, R. I., and McEwen, B. S. (1974) Oestrogen effects on brain and pituitary enzyme activities. *J. Neurochem., 23:* 925–934.

Luine, V. N., Khylchevskaya, R. I., and McEwen, B. S. (1975a) Effect of gonadal steroids on activities of monoamine oxidase and choline acetylase in rat brain. *Brain Res., 86:* 293–306.

Luine, V. N., Khylchevskaya, R. I., and McEwen, B. S. (1975b) Effect of gonadal hormones on enzyme activities in brain and pituitary of male and female rats. *Brain Res., 86:* 283–292.

Luine, V. N., and McEwen, B. S. (1977) Effects of an estrogen antagonist on enzyme activities and [³H]-estradiol nuclear binding in uterus, pituitary and brain. *Endocrinology, 100:* 903–910.

Lund, R. D., and Webster, K. E. (1967) Thalamic afferents from the spinal cord and trigeminal nuclei. An experimental anatomical study in the rat. *J. Comp. Neurol., 130:* 313–328.

Lund, S., and Pompeiano, O. (1968) Monosynaptic excitation of alpha motoneurones from supraspinal structures in the cat. *Acta Physiol. Scand., 73:* 1–21.

Lundberg, A., and Oscarsson, O. (1962) Two ascending spinal pathways in the ventral part of the cord. *Acta Physiol. Scand., 54:* 270–286.

Luttge, W. G., Gray, H. E., and Hughes, J. R. (1976) Regional and subcellular [³H] estradiol localization in selected brain regions and pituitary of female mice: effects of unlabelled estradiol and various anti-hormones. *Brain Res., 104:* 273–281.

Magoun, H. W. (1950) Caudal and cephalic influences of the brain stem reticular formation. *Physiol. Rev., 30:* 459–474.

Magoun, H. W. (1963) *The Waking Brain,* second edition. Springfield, Ill.: Thomas.

Magoun, H. W., and Rhines, R. (1946) An inhibitory mechanism in the bulbar reticular formation. *J. Neurophysiol., 9:* 165–171.

Magoun, H. W., and Rhines, R. (1947) *Spasticity: The Stretch Reflex and Extrapyramidal Systems.* Springfield, Ill.: Thomas.

Malsbury, C., Kelley, D. B., and Pfaff, D. W. (1972) Responses of single units in the dorsal midbrain to somatosensory stimulation in female rats. In C. Gaul (Ed.), *Progress in Endocrinology, Proceedings of the IV International Congress Endocrinology.* Excerpta Medica International Congress Series 273, Amsterdam: Excerpta Medica, pp. 205–209.

Malsbury, C., Kow, L.-M., and Pfaff, D. W. (1977) Effects of medial hypothalamic lesions on lordosis and other behaviors in female hamsters. *Physiol. Behav., 19:* 223–237.

Malsbury, C., and Pfaff, D. W. (1973) Suppression of sexual receptivity in the hormone-primed female hamster by electrical stimulation of the medial preoptic area. *Proc. Soc. Neurosci.,* Abstract, p. 122.

Malsbury, C., and Pfaff, D. W. (1974) Neural and hormonal determinants of mating behavior in adult male rats. A review. In L. DiCara (Ed.), *Limbic and Autonomic Nervous Systems Research.* New York: Plenum, pp. 85–136.

Malsbury, C. W. (1971) Facilitation of male rat copulatory behavior by electrical stimulation of the medial preoptic area. *Physiol. Behav., 7:* 797–805.

Malsbury, C. W. Pfaff, D. W., and Malsbury, A. M. (1980) Suppression of sexual receptivity in the female hamster: neuroanatomical projections from preoptic and anterior hypothalamic electrode sites. *Brain Res., 181:* 267–284.

Mancia, M. (1974) Mechanisms in EEG synchronization and desynchronization. XXVI International Congress of Physiological Sciences, New Delhi, Abstract, p. 46.

Manogue, K., Kow, L.-M., and Pfaff, D. W. (1980a) Lordosis in female rats following diencephalic and mesencephalic transections: role of hypothalamic–midbrain fiber connections. *Horm. Behav.,* in press.

Manogue, K., Kow, L.-M., and Pfaff, D. W. (1980b) Investigations of sensory and reflex components of lordosis behavior in the female hamster. *Horm. Behav.,* in preparation.

Martin, J. B. (1979) Brain mechanisms for integration of growth hormones secretion. *The Physiologist, 22:* 23–29.

Martin, J. R. (1976) Motivated behaviors elicited from hypothalamus, midbrain, and pons of the guinea pig (*Cavia porcellus*). *J. Comp. Physiol. Psychol., 90:* 1011–1034.

Masland, R. H., Chow, K. L., and Stewart, D. L. (1971) Receptive-field characteristics of superior colliculus neurons in the rabbit. *J. Neurophysiol., 34:* 148–156.

Matsuo, H., Arimura, A., Nair, R. M. G., and Schally, A. V. (1971) Synthesis of the porcine LH- and FSH-releasing hormone by the solid-phase method. *Biochem. Biophys. Res. Commun., 45:* 822–827.

Matsuo, H., Baba, Y., Nair, R. M. G., Arimura, A., and Schally, A. V. (1971) Structure of the porcine LH- and FSH-releasing hormone. I. The proposed amino acid sequence. *Biochem. Biophys. Res. Commun., 43:* 1334–1339.

McEwen, B., and Pfaff, D. W. (1970) Factors influencing sex hormone uptake by rat brain regions: I. Effects of neonatal treatment, hypophysectomy, and competing steroid on estradiol uptake. *Brain Res., 21:* 1–16.

McEwen, B. S., and Davis, P. G. Parsons, B., and Pfaff, D. W. (1979) The brain as a target for steroid hormone action. In W. M. Cowan, Z. W. Hall, and E. R. Kandel (Eds.), *Annu. Rev. Neurosci., 2:* 65–112.

McEwen, B. S., Denef, C. J., Gerlach, J. L., and Plapinger, L. (1974) Chemical studies of the brain as a steroid hormone target tissue. In F. O. Schmitt and F. G. Worden (Eds.), *The Neurosciences. Third Study Program.* Cambridge, Mass.: M.I.T. Press, pp. 599–620.

McEwen, B. S., Pfaff, D. W., Chaptal, C., and Luine, V. N. (1975) Brain cell nuclear retention of [^{3}H] estradiol doses able to promote lordosis: temporal and regional aspects. *Brain Res., 86:* 155–161.

McEwen, B. S., Weiss, J. M., and Schwartz, L. S. (1969) Uptake of corticosterone by rat brain and its concentration by certain limbic structures. *Brain Res., 16:* 227–241.

McEwen, B. S., Weiss, J. M. and Schwartz, L. S. (1970) Retention of corticosterone by cell nuclei from brain regions of adrenalectomized rats. *Brain Res., 17:* 471–482.

Mehler, W. R. (1969) Some neurological species differences—a posteriori. *Ann. N. Y. Acad. Sci., 167:* 424–468.

Mendell, L. M., Sassoon, E. M., and Wall, P. D. (1977) Properties of synaptic linkage from "distant" afferents onto dorsal horn neurons. *Soc. Neurosci. Abstr., 3:* 504 (Abstract 615).

Mendell, L. M., Sassoon, E. M., and Wall, P. D. (1978) Properties of synaptic linkage from long ranging afferents onto dorsal horn neurones in normal and deafferented cats. *J. Physiol. (Lond.), 285:* 299–310.

Meyer, M., LaPlante, E. S., and Campbell, B. (1960) Ascending sensory pathways from the genitalia of the cat. *Exp. Neurol., 2:* 186–190.

Meyerson, B. J., and Lindstrom, L. (1968) Effect of an oestrogen antagonist ethamoxytriphetol [MER-25] on oestrus behavior in rats. *Acta Endocrinol., 59:* 41–48.

Meyerson, B. J., and Lindstrom, L. (1973) Sexual motivation in the female rat. *Acta Physiol. Scand. (Suppl.), 389:* 1–80.

Modianos, D., Delia, H., and Pfaff, D. W. (1976) Lordosis in female rats following medial forebrain bundle lesions. *Behav. Biol., 18:* 135–141.

Modianos, D., Flexman, J. E., and Hitt, J. C. (1973) Rostral medial forebrain bundle lesions produce decrements in masculine, but not feminine, sexual behavior in spayed female rats. *Behav. Biol., 8:* 629–636.

Modianos, D., Hitt, J. C., and Flexman, J. (1974) Habenular lesions produce decrements in feminine, but not masculine, sexual behavior in rats. *Behav. Biol., 10:* 75–87.

Modianos, D., Hitt, J. C., and Popolow, H. B. (1975) Habenular lesions and feminine sexual behavior of ovariectomized rats: diminished responsiveness to the synergistic effects of estrogen and progesterone. *J. Comp. Physiol. Psychol., 89:* 231–237.

Modianos, D., and Pfaff, D. W. (1975) Facilitation of the lordosis reflex by electrical stimulation of the lateral vestibular nucleus. *Proc. Soc. Neurosci.,* Abstract 710, p. 457.

Modianos, D., and Pfaff, D. W. (1976a) Brain stem and cerebellar lesions in female rats. I. Tests of posture and movement. *Brain Res., 106:* 31–46.

Modianos, D., and Pfaff, D. W. (1976b) Brain stem and cerebellar lesions in female rats. II. Lordosis reflex. *Brain Res., 106:* 47–56.

Modianos, D., and Pfaff, D. W. (1977) Facilitation of the lordosis reflex by electrical stimulation of the lateral vestibular nucleus. *Brain Res., 134:* 333–345.

Modianos, D., and Pfaff, D. W. (1979) Medullary reticular formation lesions and lordosis reflex in female rats. *Brain Res., 171*: 334–338.

Moguilewsky, M., and Raynaud, J.-P. (1979) The relevance of hypothalamic and hyphophyseal progestin receptor regulation in the induction and inhibition of sexual behavior in the female rat. *Endocrinology, 105:* 516–522.

Monahan, M., Rivier, J., Burgus, R., Amoss, M., Blackwell, R., Vale, W., and Guillemin, R. (1971) Synthèse totale par phase solide d'un décapeptide qui stimule la sécrétion des gonadotropines hypophysaires LH et FSH. *C.R. Acad. Sci. [D] (Paris), 273:* 508–510.

Moore, R. Y. (1974) Visual pathways and the central neural control of diurnal rhythms. In F. O. Schmitt and F. G. Worden (Eds.), *The Neurosciences. Third Study Program.* Cambridge, Mass.: M.I.T. Press, pp. 537–542.

Morest, D. K. (1964) The neuronal architecture of the medial geniculate body of the cat. *J. Anat., 98:* 611–630.

Mori, S., Nishimura, H., Kurakami, C., Yamamura, T., and Aoki, M. (1978) Controlled locomotion in the mesencephalic cat: distribution of facilitatory and inhibitory regions within pontine tegmentum. *J. Neurophysiol., 41:* 1580–1591.

Morrell, J., Kelley, D., and Pfaff, D. W. (1975b) Sex steroid binding in the brains of vertebrates: studies with light microscopic autoradiography. In K. Knigge, D. Scott, H. Kobayashi, and S. Ishii (Eds.), *Brain–Endocrine Interaction,* Vol. 2. Basel: Karger, pp. 230–256.

Morrell, J., and Pfaff, D. W. (1980) Autoradiographic and histochemical comparison of estrogen-concentrating cells in ventromedial hypothalamus with neurons projecting to central grey. *Anat. Rec.,* in press.

Morrell, J., Rhodes, H., and Pfaff, D. W. (1980) Modern neuroanatomical approaches to neuroendocrine control systems. In E. Muller (Ed.), *Drugs in Neuroendocrine Control.* Amsterdam: Elsevier, in press.

Morrell, J. I., Ballin, A., and Pfaff, D. W. (1977a) Autoradiographic demonstration of the pattern of ^{3}H-estradiol concentrating cells in the brain of a carnivore, the mink, *Mustela vison. Anat. Rec., 189:* 609–624.

Morrell, J. I., Ballin, A., and Pfaff, D. W. (1977b) Topography of estrogen-accumulating cells in the brain and pituitary of the female mink. *Anat. Rec., 189:* 609–624.

Morrell, J. I., Crews, D., Ballin, A., Morgentaler, A., and Pfaff, D. W. (1979) ^{3}H-Estradiol, ^{3}H-testosterone and ^{3}H-dihydrotestosterone localization in the brain of the lizard *Anolis carolinensis:* an autoradiographic study. *J. Comp. Neurol., 188:* 201–223.

Morrell, J. I., Crews, D., Ballin, A., and Pfaff, D. W. (1977a) Autoradiographic localization of ^{3}H-estradiol, ^{3}H-testosterone and ^{3}H-dihydrotestosterone in the brain of the lizard, *Anolis carolinensis. Soc. Neurosci. Abstr.,* 352: (Abstract 1130).

Morrell, J. I., Davis, R. E., and Pfaff, D. W. (1976) Autoradiographic localization of sex steroid concentrating cells in the brain of the paradise fish after ^{3}H-estradiol or ^{3}H-testosterone administration. *Proceedings of the Fifth International Congress of Endocrinology.* Hamburg, July 1976, Abstract 278, p. 114.

Morrell, J. I., Greenberger, L. M., and Pfaff, D. W. (1978) Projections to mesencephalic central grey related to estrogenic control of reproductive behaviors. *Soc. Neurosci. Abstr., 4:* 226 (Abstract 706).

Morrell, J. I., Greenberger, L. M., and Pfaff, D. W. (1980) Projections to mesencephalic central grey related to estrogenic control of reproductive behaviors. Manuscript in preparation.

Morrell, J. I., Kelley, D. B., and Pfaff, D. W. (1975a) Autoradiographic localization of hormone-concentrating cells in the brain of an amphibian, *Xenopus laevis.* II. Estradiol. *J. Comp. Neurol., 164:* 63–78.

Moss, R. (1971) Modification of copulatory behavior in the female rat following olfactory bulb removal. *J. Comp. Physiol. Psychol., 74:* 372–382.

Moss, R. L., and Law, O. T. (1971) The estrous cycle: its influence on single unit activity in the forebrain. *Brain Res., 30:* 435–438.

Moss, R. L., and McCann, S. M. (1973) Induction of mating behavior in rats by luteinizing hormone-releasing factor. *Science, 181:* 177–179.

Moss, R. L., and McCann, S. M. (1975) Action of luteinizing hormone-releasing factor (LRF) in the initiation of lordosis behavior in the estrone-primed ovariectomized female rat. *Neuroendocrinology, 17:* 309–318.

Moss, R. L., Paloutzian, R. F., and Law, O. T. (1974) Electrical stimulation of forebrain structures and its effect on copulatory as well as stimulus-bound behavior in ovariectomized hormone-primed rats. *Physiol. Behav., 12:* 997–1004.

Mountcastle, V. B. (1974) *Medical Physiology,* Vol. 1, 13th edition. St. Louis: Mosby.

Murphy, M. R. (1974) Relative importance of tactual and nontactual stimuli in eliciting lordosis in the female golden hamster. *Behav. Biol., 11:* 115–119.

Nance, D. M., McGinnis, M., and Gorski, R. A. (1976) Interaction of olfactory and amygdala destruction with septal lesions: effects on lordosis behavior. *Soc. Neurosci. Abstr.,* p. 653: (Abstract 932).

Nance, D. M., Shryne, J., and Gorski, R. A. (1974) Septal lesions: effects on lordosis behavior and pattern of gonadotropin release. *Horm. Behav., 5:* 73–81.

Nance, D. M., Shryne, J., and Gorski, R. A. (1975) Effects of septal lesions on behavioral sensitivity of female rats to gonadal hormones. *Horm. Behav., 6:* 59–64.

Napoli, A., Powers, J. B., and Valenstein, E. (1972) Hormonal induction of behavioral estrus modified by electrical stimulation of hypothalamus. *Physiol. Behav., 9:* 115–117.

Nauta, W. J. H., and Kuypers, H. G. J. M. (1958) Some ascending pathways in the brain stem reticular formation. In H. H. Jasper, L. D. Proctor, R. S. Knighton, W. C. Noshay, and R. T. Costello (Eds.), *Reticular Formation of the Brain.* Boston: Little, Brown, pp. 3–30.

Niemer, W. T., and Magoun, H. W. (1947) Reticulo-spinal tracts influencing motor activity. *J. Comp. Neurol., 87:* 367–379.

Noble, R. G. (1972) Facilitation of the lordosis response of the female hamster (*Mesocricetus auratus*). *Physiol. Behav., 10:* 663–666.

Noble, R. G. (1973) Sexual arousal of the female hamster. *Physiol. Behav., 10:* 973–975.

Nottebohm, F., Stokes, T. M., and Leonard, C. M. (1976) Central control of song in the canary, *Serinus canaria. J. Comp. Neurol., 165:* 457–486.

Numan, M. (1974) Medial preoptic area and maternal behavior in the female rat. *J. Comp. Physiol. Psychol., 87:* 746–759.

Nyberg-Hansen, R. (1964) Origin and termination of fibers from the vestibular nuclei descending in the medial longitudinal fasciculus. An experimental study with silver impregnation methods in the cat. *J. Comp. Neurol., 122:* 355–367.

Nyberg-Hansen, R. (1965) Sites and mode of termination of reticulo-spinal fibers in the cat. An experimental study with silver impregnation methods. *J. Comp. Neurol., 124:* 71–100.

Nyberg-Hansen, R. (1966) Functional organization of descending supraspinal fibre systems to the spinal cord. Anatomical observations and physiological correlations. *Rev. Anat. Embryol. Cell Biol., 39:* 1–48.

Nyberg-Hansen, R. (1975) Anatomical aspects of the functional organization of the vestibulospinal pathways. In R. F. Naunton (Ed.), *The Vestibular System.* New York: Academic Press, pp. 71–96.

Nyberg-Hansen, R., and Mascitti, T. A. (1964) Sites and mode of termination of fibers of the vestibulospinal tract in the cat. An experimental study with silver impregnation methods. *J. Comp. Neurol., 122:* 369–387.

Parsons, B., Krieger, M., McEwen, B., and Pfaff, D. W. (1980) Long-term priming effect of estradiol on lordosis behavior in female rats. *Horm. Behav.,* in press.

Parsons, B., MacCluskey, N., Pfaff, D., and McEwen, B. S. (1980) Changes in lordosis behavior associated with hypothalamic progestin receptor content. *Endocrinology,* in press.

Paxinos, G. (1973) Midbrain and motivated behavior. *J. Comp. Physiol. Psychol., 85:* 64–69.

Paxinos, G., and Bindra, D. (1972) Hypothalamic knife cuts: effects on eating, drinking, irritability, aggression, and copulation in the male rat. *J. Comp. Physiol. Psychol., 79:* 219–229.

Peters, A., Palay, S. L., and Webster, H. deF. (1970) *Fine Structure of the Nervous System.* New York: Harper & Row.

Peterson, B. W. (1970) Distribution of neural responses to tilting within vestibular nuclei of the cat. *J. Neurophysiol.,* 1970, *33:* 750–767.

Peterson, B. W. (1979) Reticulospinal projections to spinal motor nuclei. *Ann. Rev. Physiol., 41:* 127–140.

Peterson, B. W., and Abzug, C. (1975) Properties of projections from vestibular nuclei to medial reticular formation in the cat. *J. Neurophysiol., 38:* 1421–1435.

Peterson, B. W., Anderson, M. E., and Filion, M. (1974) Responses to ponto-medullary reticular neurons to cortical, tectal and cutaneous stimuli. *Exp. Brain Res., 21:* 19–44.

Peterson, B. W., and Felpel, L. P. (1971) Excitation and inhibition of reticulos-pinal neurons by vestibular, cortical, and cutaneous stimulation. *Brain Res., 27:* 373–376.

Peterson, B. W., Filion, M., Felpel, L. P., and Abzug, C. (1975) Responses of medial reticular neurons to stimulation of the vestibular nerve. *Exp. Brain Res., 22:* 335–350.

Peterson, B. W., Maunz, R. A., Pitts, N. G., and Mackel, R. G. (1975) Patterns of projection and branching of reticulospinal neurons. *Exp. Brain Res., 23:* 333–351.

Peterson, B. W., Pitts, N. G., and Fukushima, K. (1979) Reticulospinal connec-tions with limb and axial motoneurons. *Exp. Brain Res., 36:* 1–20.

Peterson, B. W., Pitts, N. G., Fukushima, K., and Mackel, R. (1978) Reticulos-pinal excitation and inhibition of neck motoneurons. *Exp. Brain Res., 32:* 471–489.

Petras, J. M. (1967) Cortical, tectal and tegmental fiber connections in the spinal cord of the cat. *Brain Res., 6:* 275–324.

Pfaff, D. W. (1968a) Autoradiographic localization of radioactivity in the rat brain after injection of tritiated sex hormones. *Science, 161:* 1355–1356.

Pfaff, D. W. (1968b) Uptake of estradiol-17β-H^3 in the female rat brain. An autoradiographic study. *Endocrinology, 82:* 1149–1155.

Pfaff, D. W. (1970a) Mating behavior of hypophysectomized rats. *J. Comp. Physiol. Psychol., 72:* 45–50.

Pfaff, D. W. (1970b) Nature of sex hormone effects on rat sex behavior: specificity of effects and individual patterns of response. *J. Comp. Physiol. Psychol., 73:* 349–358.

Pfaff, D. W. (1973a) Interactions of steroid sex hormones with brain tissue: studies of uptake and physiological effects. In S. Segal et al. (Eds.), *The Regulation of Mammalian Reproduction.* Springfield, Ill.: Thomas, pp. 5–22.

Pfaff, D. W. (1973b) Luteinizing hormone releasing factor (LRF) potentiates lordosis behavior in hypophysectomized ovariectomized female rats. *Science, 182:* 1148–1149.

Pfaff, D. W. (1976) The neuroanatomy of sex hormone receptors in the vertebrate brain. In T. C. A. Kumar (Ed.), *Neuroendocrine Regulation of Fertility.* Basel: Karger, pp. 30–45.

Pfaff, D. W., and Conrad, L. C. A. (1978) Hypothalamic neuroanatomy: steroid hormone binding and patterns of axonal projections. In G. Bourne (Ed.), *International Review of Cytology,* Vol. 54. New York: Academic Press, pp. 245–265.

Pfaff, D. W., Diakow, C., Montgomery, M., and Jenkins, F. A. (1978) X-ray cinematographic analysis of lordosis in female rats. *J. Comp. Physiol. Psychol., 92:* 937–941.

Pfaff, D. W., Diakow, C., Zigmond, R. E., and Kow, L.-M. (1974) Neural and hormonal determinants of female mating behavior in rats. In F. O. Schmitt and F. G. Worden (Eds.), *The Neurosciences,* Vol. 3. Cambridge, Mass.: M.I.T. Press, pp. 621–646.

Pfaff, D. W., Gerlach, J., McEwen, B. S., Ferin, M., Carmel, P., and Zimmerman, E. (1976) Autoradiographic localization of hormone-concentrating cells in the brain of the female rhesus monkey. *J. Comp. Neurol., 170:* 279–294.

Pfaff, D. W., and Keiner, M. (1973) Atlas of estradiol-concentrating cells in the central nervous system of the female rat. *J. Comp. Neurol., 151:* 121–158.

Pfaff, D. W., and Lewis, C. (1974) Film analyses of lordosis in female rats. *Horm. Behav., 5:* 317–335.

Pfaff, D. W., Lewis, C., Diakow, C., and Keiner, M. (1972) Neurophysiological analysis of mating behavior responses as hormone-sensitive reflexes. In E. Stellar and J. M. Sprague (Eds.), *Progress in Physiological Psychology,* Vol. 5. pp. 253–297.

Pfaff, D. W., and Modianos, D. (1980) Neural mechanisms of female reproductive behavior. In R. Goy and D. W. Pfaff (Eds.), *Neurobiology of Reproduction.* New York: Plenum, in press.

Pfaff, D. W., Montgomery, M., and Lewis, C. (1977) Somatosensory determinants of lordosis in female rats: behavioral definition of the estrogen effect. *J. Comp. Physiol. Psychol., 91:* 134–145.

Pfaff, D. W., and Pfaffmann, C. (1969) Olfactory and hormonal influences on the basal forebrain of the male rat. *Brain Res., 15:* 137–156.

Pfaff, D. W., and Sakuma, Y. (1979a) Deficit in the lordosis reflex of female rats caused by lesions in the ventromedial nucleus of the hypothalamus. *J. Physiol., 288:* 203–210.

Pfaff, D. W., and Sakuma, Y. (1979b) Facilitation of the lordosis reflex of female rats from the ventromedial nucleus of the hypothalamus. *J. Physiol., 288:* 189–202.

Platt, J. R. (1964) Strong inference. Certain systematic methods of scientific thinking may produce much more rapid progress than others. *Science, 146:* 347–353.

Poggio, G. F., and Mountcastle, V. B. (1960) A study of the functional contributions of the lemniscal and spinothalamic systems to somatic sensibility. Central nervous mechanisms in pain. *Bull. Johns Hopkins Hosp., 106:* 266–316.

Pompeiano, O. (1975) Vestibulo-spinal relationships. In R. F. Naunton (Ed.), *The Vestibular System.* New York: Academic Press, pp. 147–184.

Pompeiano, O., and Brodal, A. (1957) Spino-vestibular fibers in the cat. An experimental study. *J. Comp. Neurol., 108:* 353–382.

Powers, B., and Valenstein, E. S. (1972) Sexual receptivity: facilitation by medial preoptic lesions in female rats. *Science, 175:* 1003–1005.

Powers, J. B. (1975) Anti-estrogenic suppression of the lordosis response in female rats. *Horm. Behav., 6:* 379–392.

Quadagno, D. M., Shryne, J., and Gorski, R. A. (1971) The inhibition of steroid-induced sexual behavior by intrahypothalamic actinomycin-D. *Horm. Behav.*, *2:* 1–10.

Raisman, G., and Brown-Grant, K. (1977) Reproductive function in male and female rats following extra- and intra-hypothalamic lesions. *Proc. Roy. Soc.* (London) *B*, *198:* 267–278.

Rhines, R., and Magoun, H. W. (1946) Brain stem facilitation of cortical motor response. *J. Neurophysiol.*, *9:* 219–229.

Robards, M. J., Watkins, D. W., III, and Masterton, R. B. (1976) An anatomical study of some somesthetic afferents to the intercollicular terminal zone of the midbrain of the opossum. *J. Comp. Neurol.*, *170:* 499–524.

Roberts, W. W., Steinberg, M. L., and Means, L. W. (1967) Hypothalamic mechanisms for sexual, aggressive, and other motivational behaviors in the opossum, *Didelphis virginiana*. *J. Comp. Physiol. Psychol.*, *64:* 1–15.

Rodgers, C. H. (1969) Total and partial surgical isolation of the male rat hypothalamus: effects on reproductive behavior and physiology. *Physiol. Behav.*, *4:* 465–470.

Rodgers, C. H., and Law, O. T. (1967) The effects of habenular and medial forebrain bundle lesions on sexual behavior in female rats. *Psychon. Sci.*, *8:* 1–2.

Rodgers, C. H., and Schwartz, N. B. (1972) Diencephalic regulation of plasma LH, ovulation, and sexual behavior in the rat. *Endocrinology*, *90:* 461–465.

Rodgers, C. H., and Schwartz, N. B. (1976) Differentiation between neural and hormonal control of sexual behavior and gonadotrophin secretion in the female rat. *Endocrinology*, *98:* 778–786.

Rose, J. D., and Sutin, J. (1973) Responses of single units in the medulla to genital stimulation in estrous and anestrous cats. *Brain Res.*, *50:* 87–99.

Rosén, I., and Scheid, P. (1973a) Patterns of afferent input to the lateral reticular nucleus of the cat. *Exp. Brain Res.*, *18:* 242–255.

Rosén, I., and Scheid, P. (1973b) Responses in the spino-reticulo-cerebellar pathway to stimulation of cutaneous mechanoreceptors. *Exp. Brain Res.*, *18:* 268–278.

Rosén, I., and Scheid, P. (1973c) Responses to nerve stimulation in the bilateral ventral flexor reflex tract (bVFRT) of the cat. *Exp. Brain Res.*, *18:* 256–267.

Ross, J. W., Paup, D. C., Brant-Zawadski, M., Marshall, J. R., and Gorski, R. A. (1973) Effects of cis- and trans-clomiphene in the induction of sexual behavior. *Endocrinology*, *93:* 681–685.

Roy, E. J., and Wade, G. N. (1977) Binding of ^{3}H-estradiol by brain cell nuclei and female rat sexual behavior: inhibition by antiestrogens. *Brain Res.*, *126:* 73–87.

Ruda, M. (1976) Autoradiographic study of the efferent projections of the midbrain central gray in the cat. Ph.D. Thesis, University of Pennsylvania. University Microfilms International, Ann Arbor, Mich.

Ruda, M. A. (1975) An autoradiographic study of the efferent connections of the midbrain central gray in the cat. *Anat. Rec.*, *181:* 468.

Ruh, T. S., and Ruh, M. E. (1974) The effect of anti-estrogens on the nuclear binding of the estrogen receptor. *Steroids*, *24:* 209–224.

Rusak, B., and Morin, L. P. (1975) Testicular responses to photoperiod are blocked by lesions of the suprachiasmatic nuclei in golden hamsters. *Soc. Neurosci. Abstr.* (Abstract 678).

Sakuma, Y., Edwards, K., and Pfaff, D. W. (1980) Role of hypothalamic periventricular fiber output in lordosis. Manuscript in preparation.

Sakuma, Y. and Pfaff, D. W. (1979a) Facilitation of female reproductive behavior from mesencephalic central grey in the rat. *Amer. J. Physiol. 237:* R278–84.

Sakuma, Y., and Pfaff, D. W. (1979b) Mesencephalic mechanisms for integration of female reproductive behavior in the rat. *Am. J. Physiol., 237:* R285–290.

Sakuma, Y., and Pfaff, D. W. (1980a) Effects of LHRH and antibody to LHRH infused in central grey on lordosis behavior in female rats. *Nature, 283:* 566–567.

Sakuma, Y., and Pfaff, D. W. (1980b) Properties of reticular and central grey mesencephalic neurons in rat, identified from lower brainstem. *J. Neurophysiol.,* in press.

Sakuma, Y., and Pfaff, D. W. (1980c) Estrogen effects on mesencephalic neurons with descending projections. *J. Neurophysiol.,* in press.

Sakuma, Y., and Pfaff, D. W. (1980d) Single unit recording from mesencephalic central grey and reticular neurons in female rats. *Exp. Neurol.,* in press.

Sawyer, C. H. (1960) Reproductive behavior. In J. Field, H. W. Magoun, and V. E. Hall (Eds.), *Handbook of Physiology. Section 1: Neurophysiology,* Vol. 2. Washington, D.C.: American Physiological Society, pp. 1225–1240.

Sawyer, C. H., and Robison, B. (1956) Separate hypothalamic areas controlling pituitary gonadotropic function and mating behavior in female cats and rabbits. *J. Clin Endocrinol. Metab., 16:* 914–915.

Schally, A. V., Baba, Y., Arimura, A. Redding, T. W., and White, W. F. (1971) Evidence for peptide nature of LH and FSH-releasing hormones. *Biochem. Biophys. Res. Commun., 42:* 50–56.

Schmidt, R. S. (1974) Neural correlates of frog calling. Trigeminal tegmentum. *J. Comp. Physiol., 92:* 229–254.

Schmitt, P., Paunovic, V. R., and Karli, P. (1979) Effects of mesencephalic central gray and raphe nuclei lesions on hypothalamically induced escape. *Physiol. Behav., 23:* 85–95.

Schneider, G. (1967) Contrasting visuomotor functions of tectum and cortex in the golden hamster. *Psychol. Forsch., 31:* 52–62.

Schneider, G. E. (1969) Two visual systems. *Science, 163:* 895–902.

Schroeder, D. M., and Jane, J. A. (1971) Projection of dorsal column nuclei and spinal cord to brainstem and thalamus in the tree shrew, *Tupaia glis. J. Comp. Neurol., 142:* 309–350.

Schwartz, N. B. (1969) A model for the regulation of ovulation in the rat. *Recent Prog. Horm. Res., 25:* 1–55.

Schwartz-Giblin, S., and Pfaff, D. W. (1980) Quantitative objective response measurements of lordosis reflex in female rats, by use of a strain gauge. *Physiology & Behavior,* in press.

Scott, J., and Pfaff, D. W. (1970) Behavioral and electrophysiological responses of female mice to male mouse urine odors. *Physiol. Behav., 5:* 407–411.

Scott, J., and Pfaffmann, C. (1967) Olfactory input to the hypothalamus: electrophysiological evidence. *Science, 158:* 1592–1594.

Scott, J. W., and Chafin, B. R. (1975) Origin of olfactory projections to lateral hypothalamus and nuclei gemini of the rat. *Brain Res., 88:* 64–68.

Sherrington, C. (1906) *The Integrative Action of the Nervous System.* New Haven: Yale University Press.

Singer, J. J. (1968) Hypothalamic control of male and female sexual behavior in female rats. *J. Comp. Physiol. Psychol., 66:* 738–742.

Skinner, B. F. (1953) *Science and Human Behavior.* New York: Macmillan.

Smalstig, E. B., and Clemens, J. A. (1975) The role of the suprachiasmatic nuclei in reproductive cyclicity. *Soc. Neurosci. Abstr.* p. 434 (Abstract 673).

Sprague, J. M., and Chambers, W. W. (1954) Control of posture by reticular formation and cerebellum in the intact, anesthetized and unanesthetized and in the decerebrated cat. *Am. J. Physiol., 176:* 52–64.

Sprague, J. M., Levitt, M., Robson, K., Liu, C. N., Stellar, E., and Chambers, W. W. (1963) A neuroanatomical and behavioral analysis of the syndromes resulting from midbrain lemniscal and reticular lesions in the cat. *Arch. Ital. Biol., 101:* 225–295.

Sprague, J. M., Schreiner, L. H., Lindsley, D. B., and Magoun, H. W. (1948) Reticulo-spinal influences on stretch reflexes. *J. Neurophysiol., 11:* 501–507.

Stein, B. E., Magalhaes-Castro, B., and Kruger, L. (1975) Superior colliculus: visuotopic–somatotopic overlap. *Science, 189:* 224–225.

Stein, B. E., Magalhaes-Castro, B., and Kruger, L. (1976) Relationship between visual and tactile representations in cat superior colliculus. *J. Neurophysiol., 39:* 401–419.

Stephan, F. K., and Zucker, I. (1972a) Circadian rhythms in drinking behavior and locomotor activity of rats are eliminated by hypothalamic lesions. *Proc. Natl. Acad. Sci. U.S.A., 69:* 1583–1586.

Stephan, F. K., and Zucker, I. (1972b) Rat drinking rhythms: central visual pathways and endocrine factors mediating responsiveness to environmental illumination. *Physiol. Behav., 8:* 315–326.

Stetson, M. H., and Watson-Whitmyre, M. (1976) Nucleus suprachiasmaticus: the biological clock in the hamster? *Science, 191:* 197–199.

Stockmeyer, L. J., and Chandra, A. K. (1979) Intrinsically difficult problems. *Sci. Am., 240:* 140–159.

Sutin, J. (1966) The periventricular stratum of the hypothalamus. *Int. Rev. Neurobiol., 9:* 263–300.

Suzuki, J.-I., and Cohen, B. (1964) Head, eye, body and limb movements from semicircular canal nerves. *Exp. Neurol., 10:* 393–405.

Szechtman, H., Caggiula, A. R., and Wulkan, D. (1975) Systematic isolation of the preoptic area with a microknife: a neuroanatomical and behavioral analysis of the disruption of sexual behavior in male rats. *Soc. Neurosci. Abstr.* p. 542 (Abstract 844).

Takeuchi, T., and Manning, J. W. (1973) Hypothalamic mediation of sinus baroreceptor-evoked muscle cholinergic dilator response. *Am. J. Physiol., 224:* 1280–1287.

ten Bruggencate, G., and Lundberg, A. (1974) Facilitatory interaction in transmission to motoneurones from vestibulospinal fibres and contralateral primary afferents. *Exp. Brain Res., 19:* 248–270.

Terasawa, E., and Sawyer, C. H. (1969) Changes in electrical activity in the rat hypothalamus related to electrochemical stimulation of adenohypophyseal function. *Endocrinology, 85:* 143–149.

Thompson, W. I. (1973) *Passages about Earth. An Exploration of the New Planetary Culture.* New York: Harper & Row, p. 124.

Tinbergen, N. (1951) *The Study of Instinct.* New York: Oxford University Press.

Valverde, F. (1962) Reticular formation of the albino rat's brain stem cytoarchitecture and corticofugal connections. *J. Comp. Neurol., 119:* 25–53.

Valverde, F. (1965) *Studies on the Piriform Lobe.* Cambridge, Mass.: Harvard University Press.

Verrier, R. L., Calvert, A., and Lown, B. (1975) Effect of posterior hypothalamic stimulation on ventricular fibrillation threshold. *Am. J. Physiol., 228:* 923–927.

Waldron, H. A., and Gwyn, D. G. (1969) Descending nerve tracts in the spinal cord of the rat. I. Fibers from the midbrain. *J. Comp. Neurol., 137:* 143–154.

Warner, R. L. (1975) Long term effects of hypothalamic deafferentation in the hamster. *Anat. Rec., 181:* 505.

Werner, G. (1974) Neural information processing with stimulus feature extractors. In F. O. Schmitt and F. G. Worden (Eds.), *The Neurosciences. Third Study Program.* Cambridge, Mass.: M.I.T. Press, pp. 171–183.

Whalen, R. E., Gorzalka, B. B., DeBold, J. F., Quadagno, D. M., Ho, G. K.-W., and Hough, J. C., Jr. (1974) Studies on the effects of intracerebral actinomycin D implants on estrogen-induced receptivity in rats. *Horm. Behav., 5:* 337–343.

Whalen, R. E., and Nakayama, K. (1965) Induction of estrous behavior: facilitation by repeated hormone treatment. *J. Endocrinol., 33:* 525–526.

Whalen, R., et al. (1980) Chapter in R. Goy and D. W. Pfaff (Eds.), *Neurobiology of Reproduction.* New York: Plenum, in press.

White, G. and Van S. (1954) Certain effects of electrolytic lesions in the hypothalamus on the mating behavior of the golden hamster. Ph.D. thesis, Louisiana State University and Agricultural and Mechanical College.

Whitehead, S. A., and Ruf, K. B. (1974) Responses of antidromically identified preoptic neurons in the rat to neurotransmitters and to estrogen. *Brain Res., 79:* 185–198.

Wickelgren, B. G. (1971) Superior colliculus: some receptive field properties of bimodally responsive cells. *Science, 173:* 69–72.

Willis, W. D., Maunz, R. A., Foreman, R. D., and Coulter, J. D. (1975) Static and dynamic responses of spinothalamic tract neurons to mechanical stimuli. *J. Neurophysiol., 38:* 587–600.

Wilson, E. O. (1975) *Sociobiology. The New Synthesis.* Cambridge, Mass.: Belknap Press of Harvard University Press.

Wilson, E. O. (1979) *On Human Nature.* London: Harvard University Press.

Wilson, V. J. (1975a) Physiology of the vestibular nuclei. In R. F. Naunton (Ed.), *The Vestibular System.* New York: Academic Press, pp. 109–128.

Wilson, V. J. (1975b) The labyrinth, the brain, and posture. *Am. Sci., 63:* 325–332.

Wilson, V. J., Kato, M., Peterson, B. W., and Wylie, R. M. (1967) A single-unit analysis of the organization of Deiter's nucleus. *J. Neurophysiol., 30:* 603–619.

Wilson, V. J., Kato, M., Thomas, R. C., and Peterson, B. W. (1966) Excitation of lateral vestibular neurons by peripheral afferent fibers. *J. Neurophysiol., 29:* 508–529.

Wilson, V. J., Uchino, Y., Susswein, A. J., and Rapoport, S. (1976) Properties of vestibular neurons projecting to the neck segments of the cat spinal cord. *Soc. Neurosci. Abstr.* p. 1055 (Abstract 1522).

Wilson, V. J., and Yoshida, M. (1969) Comparison of effects of stimulation of Deiter's nucleus and medial longitudinal fasciculus on neck, forelimb, and hindlimb motoneurons. *J. Neurophysiol., 32:* 743–758.

Wilson, V. J., Yoshida, M., and Schor, R. H. (1970) Supraspinal monosynaptic excitation and inhibition of thoracic back motoneurons. *Exp. Brain Res., 11:* 282–295.

Wuttke, W. (1974) Preoptic unit activity and gonadotropin release. *Exp. Brain Res., 19:* 205–216.

Yagi, K. (1970) Effects of estrogen on the unit activity of the rat hypothalamus. *J. Physiol. Soc. Jpn., 32:* 692–693.

Yagi, K. (1973) Changes in firing rates of single preoptic and hypothalamic units following an intravenous administration of estrogen in the castrated female rat. *Brain Res., 53:* 343–352.

Yagi, K., and Sawaki, Y. (1973) Feedback of estrogen in the hypothalamic control of gonadotrophin secretion. In K. Yagi and S. Yoshida (Eds.), *Neuroendocrine Control*. Tokyo: University of Tokyo Press, pp. 297–325.

Yamanouchi, K., and Arai, Y. (1975) Female lordosis pattern in the male rat induced by estrogen and progesterone: effect of interruption of the dorsal inputs to the preoptic area and hypothalamus. *Endocrinol. Jpn., 22:* 243–246.

Yanase, M., and Gorski, R. A. (1976) Sites of estrogen and progesterone facilitation of lordosis behavior in the spayed rat. *Biol. Reprod., 15:* 536–543.

Young, W. C. (1961) The hormones and mating behavior. In W. C. Young (Ed.), *Sex and Internal Secretions,* Vol. 2, third edition. Baltimore: Williams & Wilkins.

Young, W. C., Boling, J. L., and Blandau, R. J. (1941) The vaginal smear picture, sexual receptivity and time of ovulation in the albino rat. *Anat. Rec., 80:* 37–45.

Young, W. C., Dempsey, E. W., Hagquist, C. W., and Boling, J. L. (1937) The determination of heat in the guinea pig. *J. Lab. Clin. Med., 23:* 300–302.

Zasorin, N., Malsbury, C., and Pfaff, D. W. (1975) Suppression of lordosis in the hormone-primed female hamster by electrical stimulation of the septal area. *Physiol. Behav., 14:* 595–599.

Zemlan, F., Kow, L.-M., Morrell, J. I., and Pfaff, D. W. (1979) Descending tracts of the lateral columns of the rat spinal cord: a study using the horseradish peroxidase and silver impregnation techniques. *J. Anat., 128:* 489–512.

Zemlan, F., Kow, L.-M., and Pfaff, D. W. (1980a) Lesions of reticular and aminergic brainstem cell groups in female rats: effects on reproductive behavior and pain. *Exp. Neurol.,* in preparation.

Zemlan, F., Kow, L.-M., and Pfaff, D. W. (1980b) Noradrenergic and serotonergic effects on flexion and crossed extensor reflexes in spinal rats. *J. Pharmacol. Exp. Ther.,* in preparation.

Zemlan, F., and Pfaff, D. W. (1975) Lordosis after cerebellar damage in female rats. *Horm. Behav., 6:* 27–33.

Zemlan, F. P., Leonard, C. M., Kow, L.-M., and Pfaff, D. W. (1978) Ascending tracts of the lateral columns of the rat spinal cord: a study using the silver impregnation and horseradish peroxidase techniques. *Exp. Neurol., 62:* 298–334.

Zemlan, F. P., and Pfaff, D. W. (1979) Topographical organization in medullary reticulospinal systems as demonstrated by the horseradish peroxidase technique. *Brain Res., 174:* 161–166.

Zigmond, R. E., Detrick, R., and Pfaff, D. W. (1980) Autoradiographic localization of hormone-binding cells in the brain of the chaffinch, following administration of ^{3}H-testosterone. *Brain Res., 182:* 369–381.

Zigmond, R. E., and McEwen, B. S. (1970) Selective retention of estradiol by cell nuclei in specific brain regions of the ovariectomized rat. *J. Neurochem., 17:* 889–899.

Index